The Adaptable Mind

The Adaptable Mind

What Neuroplasticity and Neural Reuse Tell Us about Language and Cognition

JOHN ZERILLI

*Research Fellow, Cambridge University and (from 2021)
Leverhulme Trust Fellow, Oxford University*

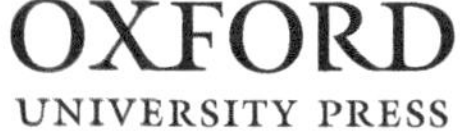

OXFORD
UNIVERSITY PRESS

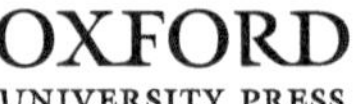

Oxford University Press is a department of the University of Oxford. It furthers the University's objective of excellence in research, scholarship, and education by publishing worldwide. Oxford is a registered trade mark of Oxford University Press in the UK and certain other countries.

Published in the United States of America by Oxford University Press
198 Madison Avenue, New York, NY 10016, United States of America.

Library of Congress Cataloging-in-Publication Data
Names: Zerilli, John, author.
Title: The adaptable mind : what neuroplasticity and neural reuse tell us about language and cognition / John Zerilli.
Description: New York : Oxford University Press, 2021. |
Includes bibliographical references and index.
Identifiers: LCCN 2020036080 (print) | LCCN 2020036081 (ebook) |
ISBN 9780190067885 (hardback) | ISBN 9780190067908 (epub) |
ISBN 9780190067915
Subjects: LCSH: Cognitive science. | Neuroplasticity. |
Language Acquisition—Psychological aspects.
Classification: LCC BF311 .Z447 2020 (print) | LCC BF311 (ebook) |
DDC 153—dc23
LC record available at https://lccn.loc.gov/2020036080
LC ebook record available at https://lccn.loc.gov/2020036081

DOI: 10.1093/oso/9780190067885.001.0001

1 3 5 7 9 8 6 4 2

Printed by Integrated Books International, United States of America

For my sister and brother, Daniela and Lucas.

Man is a machine so complicated that it is impossible at first to form a clear idea of it, and consequently to describe it. This is why all the investigations the greatest philosophers have made *a priori*, that is by wanting to take flight with the wings of the mind, have been in vain. Only *a posteriori*, by unraveling the soul as one pulls out the guts of the body, can one, I do not say discover with clarity what the nature of man is, but rather attain the highest degree of probability possible on the subject.

La Mettrie, L'Homme machine, 1748

Contents

Preface

I'd have never ventured into the field of cognitive science had it not been for the inspiring work of the linguist Noam Chomsky. I'm sure ten thousand tongues could sing this song, but whether it's a cliché or not, it's the truth. The technical brilliance, formal beauty, and extraordinary precision of his early work in transformational-generative grammar have never ceased to dazzle me. That he managed to contrive such a system while still in his twenties is simply astonishing. Anyone who has prepared a doctoral dissertation in a technical discipline knows something of the sheer brutality involved. To subvert, then reinvent, a whole technical discipline—in your twenties!—is nonpareil. I'll be forever grateful that I was able to meet him personally during his visit to Australia in November 2011. I was even fortunate enough to be able to discuss with him some of the ideas that have found their way into this book. As it happens, I have arrived at conclusions that diverge from his in significant respects. But I have not done so lightly.

A second, but equally important, source of inspiration has been the work of the cognitive neuroscientist Michael L. Anderson, whom I was also privileged to meet, this time at a workshop run by Macquarie University's Department of Cognitive Science in June 2016. The idea of neural reuse had been with me as a kind of premonition for years: indeed, from the moment I first turned away from the practice of law and began to inquire seriously into matters concerning the mind and its structure. As a 27-year-old, having never formally studied biology, linguistics, mathematics, or philosophy, I incautiously submitted a master's thesis to the University of Sydney, canvassing issues in which some knowledge of these subjects would have been advantageous (to put it mildly). It was an unmitigated disaster, and I have ever since wished to eradicate all traces of it, prevented only by the limits of my jurisdiction over the University's thesis repository. Curiously enough, I was actually awarded the degree, albeit on condition that I make a few emendations; but it was so poorly crafted and misinformed that to this day I can hardly say why. Nonetheless, and despite my embarrassment, a few ideas in the thesis stood out for being clearly articulated and not obviously implausible. One was the idea of neural reuse. Of course, I didn't call it "reuse" at the time, and had devised a rather clumsy apparatus with which to express my theoretical inklings. When I encountered Anderson's own elegantly conceived and much more skillfully executed theory of "massive redeployment," I was able to take its descriptive apparatus on board. Anderson's influence will be evident to anyone familiar with his work in the pages that follow.

A Note on my Conception of Philosophy

This is somewhat of a personal impression, but I suspect that many philosophers who work in the space around the theoretical and experimental sciences will have a similar idea of what they understand by "philosophy." As a general rule, philosophy investigates questions that cannot be satisfactorily answered by the use of either formal or axiomatic methods of inquiry (the methods of logic and mathematics), on the one hand, or by the use of empirical, scientific methods, on the other (e.g., through observation, experiment, simulation, and modeling). Thus, questions concerning the nature of knowledge—for example, regarding what we know, and how we know what we know—as well as questions concerning the ends of life—what is the good, the beautiful, and so on—are paradigms of philosophical questions. In more concrete terms, however, philosophy consists chiefly of three interrelated activities:

   (*i*)   the systematic study of concepts and schemas;
  (*ii*)   the systematic study of the presuppositions of science; and
 (*iii*)   the systematic study of values and systems of values.

I see my philosophical work here, and that of most empirically minded philosophers, as primarily engaged in the second of these activities. But as I see things, (*ii*) is really only one part of a broader endeavor that is properly called "Theoretical Science." Theoretical Science (as in Theoretical Physics, Theoretical Biology, Theoretical Linguistics, Theoretical Psychology, and so on) encompasses both the study of presuppositions in the above sense—the "Foundations of x"/the "Philosophy of x"—as well as all other scientific work that is not strictly experimental, as opposed to deductive, conjectural, or interpretative. And, truth be told, there is actually very little "Foundations of"/ "Philosophy of" going on in this book. The little that there is can certainly be described as the "Philosophy of Science," broadly, and the "Philosophy of

Cognitive Science" (or "Philosophy of Psychology"), in particular. Most of the book, however, doesn't deal with foundational concepts and presuppositions in cognitive science (e.g., "Is the computational analogy for the mind a good one?" "Are connectionist architectures better at accounting for mental operations than digital ones?" and so on). In fact, it completely sidesteps the most fundamental questions that *could* be asked of psychology (the proper purview of the "Philosophy of Mind"): for example, questions concerning the nature of the self, the relationship between mind and body, and the possibility of free will. Instead, most of the book operates at the deductive/conjectural/interpretative end of the Theoretical Science spectrum. This means that the book is more "Theoretical Psychology" than "Philosophy of Psychology," per se. My guess is that the book is about 20% Philosophy of Psychology, and 80% Theoretical Psychology.

As one might have gathered, I am sympathetic to Quine's ideas of a science–philosophy continuum, in which at one extreme, science deals with observation and verification, and at the other extreme, with conceptual difficulties. Both science and philosophy are concerned with understanding the nature of things, and both proceed by analysis and synthesis. As for which is more important, one might as well ask whether length is more important than height when calculating the area of a rectangle. Experiments never occur in a vacuum—they proceed against a background of shared and often implicit theoretical commitments, which it is the job of the philosopher to unearth and reformulate. Philosophy, for its part, needs the ballast of science to stop it from keeling over.

Acknowledgments

Special thanks are due to Kim Sterelny, Michael Anderson, Noam Chomsky, Richard Menary, Stephen Stich, Carl Craver, Colin Klein, Cecilia Heyes, Tori McGeer, Eva Jablonka, Paul Griffiths, Gualtiero Piccinini, Larry Shapiro, Tom Polger, Mark Couch, Matt Spike, Ron Planer, and Liz Irvine. Each provided support, inspiration, and encouragement one way or another, and helped me hone the arguments that form the backbone of this book.

Thanks are also due to my three friends Rebecca Riva, Jesse Hambly, and Hezki Symonds; and especially to my partner, Gavin Leuzzi, for his unfailing strength and forbearance throughout the entire process of the book's composition.

Parts of Chapter 1 are reprinted by permission from Taylor and Francis, *Philosophical Psychology*, "Against the 'system' module," by John Zerilli (copyright 2017). Parts of chapters 3, 4, and 5 are reprinted by permission from Springer Nature, *Biological Theory*, "Neural reuse and the modularity of mind: Where to next for modularity?" by John Zerilli (copyright 2019). Parts of Chapter 4 were also reprinted by permission from Taylor and Francis, *Philosophical Psychology*, "Against the 'system' module" by John Zerilli (copyright 2017). Parts of Chapter 7 (§ 7.5) were reprinted from "Neural redundancy and its relation to neural reuse" by John Zerilli (*Philosophy of Science* 86(5), 1–11; copyright 2019 by the Philosophy of Science Association; reprinted by permission from University of Chicago Press). Parts of Chapter 8 are reprinted by permission from Springer Nature, *Synthese*, "Multiple realization and the commensurability of taxonomies" by John Zerilli (copyright 2019).

The work here was supported by an Australian Government Research Training Program Scholarship.

1

Setting the Scene

A familiar trope of cognitive science, linguistics, and the philosophy of psychology over the past forty or so years has been the idea of the mind as a modular system. In the context of contemporary psychology, a modular system is typically one consisting of functionally specialized subsystems responsible for processing different classes of input, or at any rate for handling specific cognitive tasks like vision, language, logic, music, and so on. The general motivation for this idea is the belief that the mind is complex, composed of different parts that do different things—as opposed to a homogeneous whole that is indivisible and more or less uniform throughout. This "holism," which modular theories of the mind have been at pains to deny, may not, at first blush, seem like a probable contender for our best explanation of cognition: who would venture to deny that the mind is anything other than complex and intricately organized? But holism isn't quite the belief that minds are *simple*. Indeed, traditionally, holism often went along with the belief that minds are impenetrably mysterious and beyond fathoming—something like an ethereal or immaterial substance. What holism does claim, however, is that whatever it takes to make a mind, it isn't many different things, but many (or a few?) of the *same sorts* of things. Modularity can be understood as a general rejection of this claim. It avers that in order to make a mind, you're going to need many *different* sorts of things, lots of *different* moving parts.

Though no doubt a plausible, methodologically fruitful, and highly influential idea in its own right—thanks in no small part to Jerry Fodor (1983), whose pioneering effort gave it contemporary theoretical expression and substance—modularity entered the scene in a big way at just about the time that saw the arrival of a new and potentially subversive force in the behavioral and brain sciences: the mature field of neuroscience. Despite its earlier beginnings, neuroscience only really came of age in the late twentieth century, and one of its outstanding achievements has been the discovery of the brain's lifelong powers of renewal and reorganization. Neuroplasticity has, for better or worse, challenged many of the orthodox conceptions of the mind that originally led cognitive scientists to postulate mental modules. Similarly,

The Adaptable Mind. John Zerilli, Oxford University Press (2021). © Oxford University Press.
DOI: 10.1093/oso/9780190067885.003.0001

rapidly accumulating neuroscientific evidence of the reuse or redeployment of neural circuits, revealing the integrated and interactive structure of brain regions, has upset basic assumptions about the relationship of function to structure upon which modularity—not to say neuroscience itself—originally depended. These movements, developments, and cross-currents are the subject of this book.

Although there are many reasons one might find the "modularity of mind" an interesting hypothesis, an especially compelling one is the possibility that it could account for our linguistic abilities. Indeed, the notion that language is not just phylogenetically special—unique to the human species—but also *cognitively* special—unique within the overall envelope of our cognitive talents—makes the modularity of mind a wonderfully intriguing hypothesis. Noam Chomsky (1975, p. 4) once remarked that "[t]o come to know a human language would be an extraordinary intellectual achievement for a creature not specifically designed to accomplish this task." If by "specifically designed" he meant "equipped with a special-purpose faculty of the mind," it is just this claim that I wish to dissect in this book. Many cognitive scientists continue to believe that language is cognitively special, and hence that its operating principles cannot be assimilated to the rules or procedures engaged within other domains of cognition (such as general problem-solving or pattern recognition). As Annette Karmiloff-Smith (1994, p. 698) once vividly expressed this point: "Lining up objects does not form the basis of word order. Trying to fit one toy inside another has nothing to do with embedded clauses." The issue is tied up in what is possibly the most contentious and acrimonious dispute in all of modern linguistics: Is language innately specified?

Throughout this book, I shall be concerned predominantly with the following question: Could something having the rough outlines of Jerry Fodor's module account for language processing? And if not, what sort of module might plausibly take its place, if any? It will be my contention that language is *not* subserved by a module in Fodor's sense, at least not in a straightforward way, and this makes *that* notion misleading as far as language modules go. I shall argue from principles of both neural reuse and neural redundancy that language is facilitated by a composite of modules (or module-like entities), none of which is likely to be linguistically special, and that neuroplasticity provides evidence that few of them ought to be considered developmentally robust, though their development seems to be definitely constrained by features intrinsic to particular regions of cortex.

There is a conspicuous lack of consensus surrounding the status of modules as neuroanatomical entities, in part because modularity has proven itself to be a highly versatile concept, sustaining different research agendas across the biological and mind sciences. Are they functionally dedicated, innately designated (species-constant) regions of "wetware" whose operations may be described by algorithms (Quartz & Sejnowski 1994, p. 726); or are they in the nature of "software" systems having no phylogenetically necessary relation to specific cortical sites, be they dedicated or otherwise? Is there indeed room for both types, or for hybrids combining features of both types (Horst 2011, pp. 224–225, 261–262)? Fodor, perhaps sensing that the real interest of modules lies partly in their functional/neural dedication and ontogenetic robustness, considered that the first description could serve as a paradigm of modularity—a view that has the merit of being in broad agreement with the neurosciences (Bechtel & Mundale 1999; Anderson & Finlay 2014, p. 5; but cf. Doidge 2007, pp. 291–297; Gold & Roskies 2008, p. 354; see §§ 4.2–4.3, this volume, for further detail). Nevertheless, in recent decades, enthusiasts of modularity have been more willing to throw their lot in with alternative proposals or otherwise endorse increasingly anodyne suggestions about what a module really amounts to. Apart from the general explosion of discoveries in the neurosciences, new and dramatic evidence of the precise extent of neuroplasticity and neural reuse has necessitated a shift of emphasis away from implementation. The innateness hypothesis alone looks to be disastrously discredited if the potential for neuroplasticity is indeed as advanced as it appears, since it underscores the crucial role that learning must play in the acquisition of competencies otherwise presumed fixed or defined by characteristic ontogenetic pace and sequencing. The evidence of neural reuse, for its part, indicates that high-level cognitive tasks such as language processing are enabled by highly distributed neural networks composed of very many smaller brain regions or nodes that are themselves multifunctional and domain-general: the selfsame circuits are redeployed over and over again across different tasks and task categories. This discovery potentially undermines the claim that such high-level cognitive feats reflect domain-specific competencies. Quandaries like these have understandably motivated the attempt to rescue the theory through a renewed emphasis on computational design (Jungé & Dennett 2010; Anderson 2010; Anderson & Finlay 2014, p. 5).

Here I shall take as my guiding idealization something closer to Fodor's paradigm of modularity, the simple reason being that it has by far been the most influential account of faculty psychology in recent decades and the one that overwhelmingly animates, or at least frequently situates, discussions concerning the modularity of language (Chomsky 1980a, pp. 39, 44; 1988, p. 159; 2002, pp. 84–86; Plaut 1995; Pinker & Jackendoff 2005, p. 207; Fitch et al. 2005, p. 182; Collins 2008, p. 155; Fedorenko & Thompson-Schill 2014; see also Karmiloff-Smith 1992). In its neurophysiological and neuroanatomical respects, Fodor's paradigm module also closely resembles the notion of a brain module familiar to the neurosciences (see Chapter 4). Thus I take a "module" to be something more substantial than a mere "cognitive system." Specifically, I take a module to be a specialized and autonomous cognitive mechanism that is reliably associated with a unique neural structure, whether local or distributed.[1] As far as I can see, only a proposal along these lines has any chance of making modularity interesting and worth pursuing. I take the possibility of functional decomposition—the possibility of understanding a complex subject by breaking it down into different "parts" (regardless of whether these "parts" overlap in the brain)—as being uncontroversial: *of course* a domain needs to be broken down if we are to have any hope of gaining insights into how it functions! So those insisting that language is modular because it furnishes a fruitful "domain of inquiry" don't collect any prizes in my book (see § 4.2.3). If I were pressed to stipulate necessary and sufficient conditions, I would lay down functional specificity (i.e., dissociability in principle) as the *sine qua non* of modularity (Carruthers 2006; Barrett & Kurzban 2006). I explain and defend this position in Chapter 4.

In the interests of full disclosure, let me stress that, by "autonomous," I do not mean automatic, autonomic, or mandatory; i.e., reflexive (rather than *reflective*) and therefore independent from central decision and control. I have a somewhat broader notion in mind, with automaticity representing only an especially extreme case. A system in my usage is autonomous when it can even moderately perform without conscious advertence, just as "skills that are practiced over and over acquire a certain degree of autonomy and insularity" (Ohlsson 1994, p. 224). An experienced pianist who does not deliberate over the arpeggios in a well-rehearsed performance, or who holds a conversation as she plays; even a driver holding a conversation as she shifts gears—each capacity displays a measure of autonomy from central control (Rasmussen 1986; Stanton & Salmon 2009; Walker et al. 2015). The

---

[1] I construe the term "structure" here quite loosely, potentially including ion channels and receptors.

operation is still subject to the will, and therefore not quite *out* of control, but it runs on autopilot all the same.[2] Actually, the examples of the pianist and the driver juggling more than one task, with one of the tasks running autonomously, share their juggling-act-like characteristics with language parsing and speech production. Fluent reading, too, where the process of instant character recognition runs autonomously of textual comprehension, is yet another example of information processing sharing features with expert musicianship, fine multitasking motor control, and language parsing (although of course reading, unlike language parsing, requires explicit instruction and drilling). Notice that these observations are consistent with the possibility that at least some modules are "made, not born" (Bates 1999). Often the claim is made that truly interesting modules are innate. But I follow most theorists in regarding innateness as a merely contingent rather than essential feature of modularity (e.g., Coltheart 1999), interesting though it certainly would be if a module were innate (see p. 7).

On the other hand, by "specialized" or "dedicated," I shall mean more or less what Fodor means when he describes modules as informationally encapsulated, domain-specific, functionally dissociable, and neurally localized. "Informational encapsulation" refers to a module's restricted access to information outside its own system-specific data store (e.g., a visual module's being impervious to beliefs the agent has about what she is seeing[3]), while "domain specificity" refers to a module's sensitivity to a restricted domain of inputs (e.g., visual, auditory, grammatical, etc.; see the discussion in §§ 2.4.3 and 5.1 for a clarification—and restatement—of this principle). A system is dissociable if it handles a specific function that can be selectively impaired, as when damage to a specific region of the brain causes a selective deficit (e.g., when speech comprehension is impaired, but speech production is not). Finally, a system is localized when it is uniquely subserved by relatively circumscribed or contiguous neural circuitry (Fodor 1983, p. 99; Prinz 2006; Robbins 2009; Gerrans 2014, p. 46). Actually, there is no cogent reason to believe that a module has to be contained within the topographical limits of a specific neural site—its processing parts could well be scattered over the whole cortex, or indeed the whole brain. So the main point of my calling

---

[2] Independence from central decision and control is a concomitant of independence from central information (or "cognitive impenetrability"), a special kind of "informational encapsulation" (see next paragraph).

[3] This is but one instance of informational encapsulation, often referred to as "cognitive impenetrability." In general, when I use the term "informational encapsulation," I mean it in the broadest sense, not in the limited sense denoting cognitive impenetrability alone.

attention to this last feature is to remind the reader that a module has to be *exclusively* realized somewhere in the brain, even if this "somewhere" is not contiguous.

For convenience, we can refer to a specialized module as an "anatomical" module (Bergeron 2007; Anderson 2010). Occasionally it will be necessary to use the term "specialized" in a somewhat stricter sense than applies to anatomical modules. Specialization in this stricter sense refers to non-reusability across multiple domains, which is essentially a very rigid kind of domain specificity. The clearest examples of units specialized in this stronger sense would be the constituent elements of an anatomical module: the dedication of modular elements to their parent module renders them dedicated or specialized in a strict sense. The parent module will be specialized in a loose sense of the word at least—specialized in the sense that it does some functionally discrete thing, and presumably the *same* thing every time; but if the parent is reusable across multiple cognitive domains, it will not be specialized in the stricter sense I have in mind (see § 5.1 for an extended discussion).

Now, while the foregoing notion of modules suffices to furnish a general target of inquiry, there are only two features of such modules to which I shall be drawing special attention in this book; namely, *functional dissociability* and *innateness*. As I have already foreshadowed, I shall argue that dissociability is the *sine qua non* of modularity (Chapter 4). This focus at once emphasizes that a module is a special-purpose, special-structure device: to the extent that separately modifiable cognitive systems exist, it is because there are *to that extent* separately modifiable neural processes. The more the neural hardware is shared (or "reused") as between distinct cognitive functions, the less likely will such functions be selectively modifiable (barring some principle of neural plasticity or compensation). Presumably, if *all* the relevant neural structures (circuits, pathways, ions, etc.) were reused across *all* cognitive functions, cognitive dissociations would not be possible. Such a conclusion seems extreme, but it is implicit even in the view of those who maintain that dissociations are compatible with pervasive neural reuse. Ritchie and Carruthers (2010, p. 289), for example, state that "at the limit, two modules could share *all* of their processing parts while still remaining dissociable and separately modifiable. For the differences might lie entirely in the patterns of connectivity among the parts, in such a way that those connections could be separately disrupted or improved." This is plausible,[4]

---

[4] But see my § 5.2.

and implicit in the conjecture is that *some* structure (even if it is just the connection pathway between two circuits) must be unique to a function in order for that function to be dissociable at all.

As for the focus on innateness, my defense is that, especially in linguistics, a traditionally very powerful argument for the modularity of linguistic abilities makes much of the fact that language acquisition in children proceeds in a breathtakingly effortless fashion, and in the face of frequently degenerate input. That is, the developmental schedule of language in most normal, healthy children unfolds at such a pace and in such a fashion as to suggest that children are, in Chomsky's words, "specifically designed to accomplish this task." I accept that language acquisition in children is impressive, but to make my case in this book, I'll need to consider whether, even if language acquisition is as effortless and speedy as has been alleged, this developmental phenomenon really does force us back into the arms of modularity. So innateness will join dissociability in my examination of the subject.

Perhaps unsurprisingly, these two features together also typify what seems to be a sort of defeasible starting position in many discussions of modularity (see, e.g., the observations by Barrett & Kurzban 2006, pp. 638, 641; Bergeron 2007)[5] and are prominent within the accounts of those defending the existence of a language module.[6] In addition, they offer an ideal segue into discussions concerning such functional characteristics as encapsulation and domain specificity (see Fedorenko & Thompson-Schill 2014, and Anderson & Finlay 2014, p. 4; also note Chomsky 1975, pp. 40–41). I'll explain why this is the case as we go along. At any rate, these are the properties I'll be evaluating in the light of evidence of neuroplasticity and neural reuse, pursuing the implications of such exciting new discoveries in neuroscience for our understanding of the modularity of mind and language in particular. The aim is to explore candidly what such discoveries suggest about the existence of modules in the robust sense I take to be interesting.

The structure of the book is as follows: Chapters 2 and 3 provide an overview of both neuroplasticity and neural reuse in the human brain. The brain

---

[5] Peter Carruthers (2006, p. 2): "In the weakest sense, a module can just be something like: a dissociable functional component." Admittedly, some, indeed Fodor himself, have nominated other properties such as encapsulation as the *sine quibus non* of modularity.

[6] In most cases, the precise notion of a "language module" at stake is somewhat more fine-grained than this crude description might initially suggest, contemplating such distinct varieties as both Fodor's sentence parser and the broad language faculty that encompasses Chomsky's Merge (see my Chapter 7). Notice that in Chomsky's usage, the terms language "organ," "faculty," "module," and "acquisition device" are used interchangeably (see, e.g., Chomsky 1980a, pp. 39, 44; 1988, p. 159; 2002, pp. 84–86).

exhibits quite remarkable plasticity. I explore various forms of plasticity, of which synaptic plasticity is perhaps the most important, given its likely role in the formation of cortical maps. This chapter concludes with a brief examination of a special kind of cortical map reorganization; namely, supramodal plasticity. This leads directly on to the notion of neural reuse, which I survey in Chapter 3.

Chapters 4 through 6 pursue the implications of neural reuse and plasticity for the modularity of mind. Chapter 4 presents an overview of the history of modular theorizing about the mind, and uses this historical context to present various conceptions of modularity. I argue against soft conceptions of modularity, and defend dissociability as the *sine qua non* of modularity. Chapter 5 considers the implications of neural reuse, while Chapter 6 considers the implications of neuroplasticity. Chapter 7 then considers the implications of both neural reuse and neuroplasticity for language. Chapter 8 rounds off the argument by casting doubt on the empirical claim that psychological states are multiply realized. The aim of this chapter is to refute the idea that cognitive science cannot be constrained by neuroscience, an idea that has regrettably obstructed fruitful collaboration between neuroscience and psychology in the past and that could prove to be even more damaging in the future, when evidence of neural reuse looks set to make things a whole lot more interesting. I conclude with some final reflections in Chapter 9.

2
Aspects of Neuroplasticity

2.1 Scope of Chapter

This chapter reviews the general science of neuroplasticity with a focus on those aspects of relevance to the modularity of mind. The need for such a review stems ultimately from an interest in the implications of neuroplasticity, particularly for the understanding of early development. While not enough is known about the molecular and cellular mechanisms underpinning neuroplasticity to warrant definite conclusions about development, tentative suggestions, grounded firmly in the available evidence, can and should be put forward. These form the subject of Chapter 6. The present chapter provides for the most part only a précis of the evidence as it stands.

2.2 The Nature of Plastic Changes in the Brain

2.2.1 Definition

Learning raises an interesting question for the cognitive and neural sciences. On one hand, the nervous system appears to be wired very precisely. On the other hand, mammalian and especially human behavior can be extremely flexible. If connections between the main signaling units of the nervous system are set during early development, how is it that behavior and its neural underpinnings can be flexible at all? What is the extent of neural fixity and flexibility in early development, and how is it related to the stability and dynamism exhibited under different conditions in later life (e.g., during learning or rehabilitation)? The best answer so far attempted and empirically substantiated is the plasticity hypothesis (Kandel et al. 2013, p. 37). This recognizes what for most of the twentieth century was denied: that even after a critical period in early childhood, the brain retains its plastic potential throughout life. It appears that "chemical synapses are functionally and anatomically modified through experience and learning as much as during

The Adaptable Mind. John Zerilli, Oxford University Press (2021). © Oxford University Press.
DOI: 10.1093/oso/9780190067885.003.0002

early development" (Kandel et al. 2013, p. 37). Plasticity is an intrinsic and persistent property of the nervous system without which it would be impossible to understand normal psychological function, or indeed pathological and contrapathological responses to events throughout life (Pascual-Leone et al. 2005, p. 378). Plasticity is not to be conceived of as an occasional or exceptional state of the nervous system—it is in fact its normal and ongoing condition (Pascual-Leone et al. 2005, p. 379). What is more, similar mechanisms appear to be at work in both adult plasticity and early development, suggesting that the mechanisms of adult learning and developmental plasticity are to some considerable extent conserved (Saitoe & Tully 2001; Kolb et al. 2001, p. 224; Neville & Bavelier 2001, p. 261). This last point is crucial, since it is really only by virtue of such parallels that adult neuroplasticity can serve as a window onto early developmental processes and carry significance for traditional debates in psychology; for example, about the innateness of language. As Laurence and Margolis observe:

> Widespread and significant instances of neural plasticity suggest an inherent openness to the functions that any cortical area can take on. If this is right, then the brain's concept acquisition capacities needn't be innately constrained toward any particular outcome. Instead cortical circuits might simply form as required to accommodate a learner's needs given whatever contingent sensory input has been received and the wiring that has been previously established. (2015, p. 124)

Neuroplasticity has been defined as "a change (either a strengthening or weakening) in synaptic efficacy brought about through experience" (Rose & Rankin 2001, p. 176). In fact, synaptic plasticity is only one of a family of brain plasticities falling under the general banner of neuroplasticity. In its widest sense, "neuroplasticity" refers simply to "the capacity of the nervous system to modify its organization," especially in response to experience, and includes the varied circumstances of normal development and maturation, learning in both immature and mature organisms, recovery of function after injury, and compensation following sensory deprivation (Neville & Bavelier 2001, p. 261). At the same time, neuroplasticity transverses *every* level of organization in the brain, synaptic events having counterparts in both higher and lower levels of organization, running all the way from genes right through to complex behavior (Shaw & McEachern 2001). These facts should not, of course, be taken to suggest that a synaptic definition of neuroplasticity is necessarily mistaken. Indeed, it is just because the synaptic level continues to provide the best understood and arguably most powerful model of neuroplasticity available—synaptic plasticity has a probable role in all of the developmental stages just described, for instance—that it has become customary to regard synaptic plasticity as broadly representative of the phenomenon. Given my concern with modules and the likely role of synaptic plasticity in the arrangement and rearrangement of cortical circuitry (Neville & Bavelier 2001, p. 261; Shaw & McEachern 2001, p. 434), there is actually good reason for framing the discussion of neuroplasticity here in terms of synaptic plasticity. Synaptic plasticity supplies a familiar and tractable neurobiological model for understanding the cases of neuroplasticity that are likely to be of direct concern to the modularity of mind; namely, cortical reorganization and memory consolidation. Still, it is important to appreciate that the term "neuroplasticity" has a significantly wider scope than the plasticity associated with merely one level of the brain's organization; and after a brief treatment of synaptic plasticity revealing the mechanisms underlying plastic change, I must ultimately turn to consider cortical map reorganization—an instance of neuroplasticity that ought to be prioritized in any serious discussion of modularity (Rowland & Moser 2014). (As for the relationship between modules and cortical maps, see the discussion in § 4.3.)

2.2.2 Synaptic plasticity

Neurons are the basic cellular units of the nervous system—self-sufficient, specialized cells whose primary function is to receive, integrate, and transmit information throughout the body. Any neuron will receive information from potentially many thousands of other neurons through a "synapse"—a cleft between the terminals ("axons") and receptive fibers ("dendrites") of adjacent neurons. Neural connections may be strengthened or weakened in a variety of ways, but the most frequently cited mechanism involves adjustments to the quantity of neurotransmitter released from the presynaptic cell and/or the number of postsynaptic receptors, which determine how effectively the postsynaptic cell can respond to the quantity of neurotransmitter released presynaptically. Strengthening occurs typically by persistent stimulation of the postsynaptic cell. A neurotransmitter's release into the synaptic cleft initiates a cascade of biochemical events that may lead to the excitation (or "potentiation") of the postsynaptic neuron.

Research has repeatedly turned up a number of neurotransmitters, neuromodulators, and ions that appear to be crucial for synaptic plasticity, including glutamate and calcium ions (Ca^{++}). Glutamate is among the most excitatory of neurotransmitters so far discovered and works by inducing a postsynaptic calcium influx, which, through repeated stimulation, may result in an action potential. More precisely, the influx of Ca^{++} leads to increases in the number and efficacy of postsynaptic α-amino-3-hydroxy-5-methyl-4-isoxazolepropionic acid (AMPA) receptors, themselves crucial for consolidating synaptic connections by providing the primary excitatory input drive on the postsynaptic neuron.

Initially, synaptic plasticity was thought to be limited to such molecular mechanisms alone, entailing few if any changes to the shape of dendritic spines or the number of axonal branches and sprouts (i.e., neuromorphological changes leading to "synaptogenesis" and synaptic "pruning"—the establishment of new connections and elimination of existing connections), while "neurogenesis" (the generation of new neurons) was understood to be an exclusively developmental process. It is now known that beyond enhanced signaling between neurons, synaptic plasticity routinely involves changes to neuromorphology, and that neurogenesis occurs well into adult life, not just perinatally as was once thought (Rose & Rankin 2001, p. 176; Fuchs & Flügge 2014).[1]

Two varieties of plasticity widely considered to involve changes at the synapse are *cortical map plasticity* (otherwise known as *representational* or *topographic map plasticity*) and the cellular changes attendant on learning and memory consolidation (Buonomano & Merzenich 1998). "Cortical map plasticity" refers to the detailed remodeling of cortical maps in response to "behaviourally important experiences throughout life" (Buonomano & Merzenich 1998, p. 150). Evidenced across different modalities in a significant number of mammalian species, including humans, cortical map reorganization not only results from behavioral changes, the environment, and injury in later life, but is at least partly responsible for some kinds of early perceptual and motor learning (Buonomano & Merzenich 1998, p. 150). It covers language cross-lateralization (migration of function from the left to the right hemisphere) following injury or trauma early in life (and even later in life, with adequate

---

[1] Cf. Sorrells et al. (2018), who conclude that adult hippocampal neurogenesis is "extremely rare" in humans.

rehabilitative training), as well as, perhaps most especially, the plasticity of sensory and motor maps in response to use or trauma. Notice that in the context of cortical map plasticity it becomes more useful to think of plasticity as the opening and closing (or broadening and narrowing) of afferent input channels. It is this plasticity that seems to have most recently captivated philosophers (see further discussion at § 8.2.2.1).

While the cellular changes involved in learning and memory consolidation are *also* thought to depend on synaptic plasticity, it has been far from easy obtaining empirical confirmation of this connection, or indeed of whether the same plastic mechanisms are involved in both cortical map plasticity and memory-related synaptic plasticity (Buonomano & Merzenich 1998, p. 150). Mainstream opinion in the field seems to err on the side of an affirmative connection on both counts (Buonomano & Merzenich 1998, pp. 152, 153), but Buonomano and Merzenich (1998, p. 179, cf. p. 165) cautiously conclude that, as for the connection between synaptic plasticity and cortical map plasticity, "we do not yet have a sufficient understanding of synaptic and cellular plasticity to fully account for the experimental data on cortical representational reorganization."

The kind of memory involved is important to clarify here. There are generally two broad classes of memories distinguished by psychologists. The first is known as "explicit" or "declarative" memory, which in turn consists of both "episodic" memory for events and "semantic" memory for concepts and facts. The second class is known as "implicit" memory, which is what could be considered the memory for *actions*. An important class of implicit memories, relating specifically to learned skills and habits, is called "procedural" memory—on account of its role in the performance of routine procedures involving neither deliberation nor specific memories of having carried them out previously (e.g., brushing one's teeth, tying one's shoelaces, riding a bicycle, etc.). Procedural memory is in effect the memory for automated action cued by specific contexts and stimuli.

While models of memory-related synaptic plasticity certainly can (and perhaps do) explain the neurophysiology of explicit memory consolidation (especially semantic memory), it is implicit and procedural memory that is perhaps their more natural target (Rose & Rankin 2001, p. 176). For one thing, procedural memory is plausibly more likely to reflect the neurophysiology of learning and memory than is something like episodic memory, which is somewhat difficult to construe in terms of the establishment and maintenance of synaptic connections. In contrast, procedural memory epitomizes the rule that "practice makes perfect," making it the more obvious candidate for explanation in terms of altered connection strengths arising from persistent, repeated cellular activation. It is also worth noting that the theory of procedural memory answers a set of concerns similar to those addressed by the theory of modularity, which in its Fodorian guise was likewise put forward to explain targeted and automated behavior involving interconnected cortical networks.

The clearest case of synaptic plasticity, and one that is likely to play some role in, or otherwise serve as a model for, memory consolidation—and possibly many other varieties of neuroplasticity—is hippocampal long-term potentiation (LTP), which, as its name suggests, is the enduring association of neurons through repeated afferent activation in the hippocampal formation. While its role in learning and memory is not conclusively established, some such role has been conjectured to exist from its resemblance to "Hebbian plasticity," named after the Canadian psychologist D. O. Hebb. Hebb's (1949) influential model of plasticity was advanced to explain the long-lasting changes in synaptic strength that he hypothesized to underlie learning and memory. He assumed that stable changes in synaptic efficacy could occur through interactions among neurons:

> When an axon of cell A is near enough to excite a cell B and repeatedly or persistently takes part in firing it, some growth process or metabolic change takes place in one or both cells such that A's efficacy, as one of the cells firing B, is increased. (1949, p. 62)

Hebb's postulate asserts that simultaneous or rapidly successive pre- and postsynaptic activity results in a strengthened connection between cells ("cells that fire together wire together; cells that fire apart wire apart," as it is often put). This requires a "coincidence detector" that records the co-concurrent or rapidly successive activity of pre- and postsynaptic neurons (Buonomano & Merzenich 1998, p. 154). In hippocampal LTP, a subtype of the glutamate receptor, so-called N-methyl-D-aspartate (NMDA) receptor, serves this coincidence-detecting function by facilitating the postsynaptic influx of Ca^{++} (which, if persistent, typically results in a strengthened connection via increased AMPA receptor efficacy, as we saw earlier). Since LTP appears to reflect something like Hebbian associative plasticity, many neuroscientists have not hesitated in postulating LTP as the neurochemical basis of learning and memory. It has the unique phenomenology, induction characteristics, and longevity "to place it firmly as a candidate for the storage of experiential memory" (Teyler 2001, p. 101).[2]

While LTP is generally regarded as crucial to memory storage, some neuroscientists are more circumspect, either denying that the evidence of LTP's subserving learning and memory is strong enough to justify the faith placed in this mechanism (Cain 2001, p. 126), or maintaining that LTP might instead be "a generic mechanism for increasing synaptic gain throughout the brain whenever increases in synaptic strength are needed," and therefore "a general purpose mechanism by which synapses can increase their influence . . . regardless of the kind of circuit in which they are embedded" (Teyler 2001, p. 105). An equally pessimistic estimate has it that "if LTP occurs naturally in the behaving animal, it can at best be said to underlie *circuit* formation, not learning or memory" (Shaw & McEachern 2001, p. 434). LTP may then, on a minimal reading, simply be a means by which neural networks are formed and maintained. But what few would deny is that LTP is an important neurophysiological substrate supporting various manifestations of neuroplasticity.[3] In fact, if the connection between implicit memory and modules is rightly drawn, LTP, even in a deflationary view, could be seen as offering support to the idea that similar synaptic mechanisms are implicated in the consolidation of memory, the development of modules, and the migration of cortical maps, which, like memories and modules, are also represented in stable, if more local, networks of neurons in the brain. (Rowland & Moser [2014] present evidence that even episodic memory has modular organization, resembling the neuroanatomical and neurophysiological features of sensory and motor cortical maps, such as columnar structure and topographic arrangement. See §§ 2.4 and 4.3 for elaboration.)

2.3 Neuroplastic Recovery During Development

While critical-period plasticity may under the right set of circumstances be "reopened" in later life, the potential for plastic recovery following injury is still very much a function of age. During development, so-called spontaneous changes to the brain resulting from injury are likely overall

---

[2] There is evidence that cortical LTP shares many of its properties with hippocampal LTP (Buonomano & Merzenich 1998, pp. 157, 174).

[3] The same could be said for long-term depression.

to reduce the plasticity of the region affected; "[i]n contrast, when the brain fails to change in response to injury there is considerable capacity for modification of cortical circuitry," particularly through experience, and here the general rule seems to be that the earlier the injury and therapeutic intervention, the better the chance of functional recovery (Kolb et al. 2001, pp. 236–237, 239). This is ostensibly because earlier interventions influence spontaneous changes "in such a way as to maximize functional recovery." On the whole, younger animals are more plastic than older ones, when it comes to both experience- or activity-dependent learning and spontaneous recovery from injury (Shaw & McEachern 2001, p. 430).

The developing brain is obviously different at different stages, so the character of spontaneous responses to injury can naturally be expected to differ with age. (Whether these responses are beneficial will also depend on age.) The best-studied case of mammalian plasticity is probably in the rat. Neurogenesis in the rat is essentially complete by birth and produces a cortex that is initially equipotential. Between seven and ten days of age, the process of cell migration in the cortex—a process that begins well before birth—comes to an end, at which point activity-independent cell differentiation begins. This process itself ends by about 15 days of age (i.e., at about the time of eye opening), although synaptogenesis continues for a further two to three weeks beyond this point. Compensation for injury suffered during neurogenesis can be quite extensive (Kolb et al. 2001, pp. 228–229). Even the killing of *all* cerebral neurons by X-radiation appears to provoke regeneration resulting in up to 50 percent of the cerebrum being rebuilt (Kolb et al. 2001, p. 229). Injuries occurring during the period of cell migration and differentiation, however, are functionally devastating, with effects even more pronounced than those caused by the same injuries in adult rats. Then again, during the period immediately following this—and therefore concurrent with a period of intense synaptogenesis—the brain's capacity for recovery seems to be optimal (Kolb et al. 2001, p. 230).

Just why young neurons are more plastic than older ones is unclear, but a very plausible hypothesis attributes it to the impact of homeostatic mechanisms after the critical period (Shaw & McEachern 2001, pp. 443–444). The absence of homeostatic regulatory mechanisms (like lateral inhibition) during critical periods means that potentiation is ubiquitous and the central nervous system highly unstable. Later, however, homeostatic regulation of receptors and synapses becomes paramount, and lateral inhibition becomes a dominant feature of neural circuits and the interaction between systems. Given such mechanisms of global homeostasis, the alterations that do occur in the adult CNS [*central nervous system*] only do so in response to the strongest stressors. (Shaw & McEachern 2001, pp. 443–444)

One upshot of this explanation is that, in one sense, the brain remains intrinsically as plastic as ever, its plastic potential merely suppressed by mechanisms that can themselves be reversed, as we now know they can, "under precisely defined and controlled conditions."

2.4 Cortical Map Plasticity

2.4.1 Intramodal plasticity

The most convincing evidence of cortical map plasticity comes from studies of plastic changes to adult primary sensory cortices. Sensory cortical areas relating to touch, vision and hearing "all represent their respective epithelial surfaces in a topographic manner" (Buonomano & Merzenich 1998, p. 152). This means neighboring cortical areas respond to neighboring sensory receptors. Somatosensory cortex maps areas of the skin's surface somatotopically such that "neighboring cortical regions respond to neighboring skin sites." Likewise, auditory cortices map tones tonotopically, and visual cortices map features of the visual field retinotopically. Close to three decades of research now confirm the potential for these sensory cortices, and their somatotopic, tonotopic, and retinotopic coordinates to undergo plastic changes in a use-dependent manner (Buonomano & Merzenich 1998, p. 152).

The plastic changes in view here could well include the recovery of function after injury to the cortex; for example, language cross-lateralization following trauma (Polger 2009, p. 464; Clark 2009, p. 365). In such cases, a certain psychological function, be it tactile, visual, auditory, motor, or linguistic, is mediated by a specific region of cortex at time t_1, and by a different region of cortex at time t_2 (Polger 2009, p. 464). A particularly striking example of this is seen in the case of children who develop normal or nearly normal language abilities after a left hemispherectomy, in which the left cerebral hemisphere (which typically mediates language) is either disabled or removed in its entirety (Laurence & Margolis 2015, p. 123). A child known as "EB" was found to have recovered most of his language skills two years after undergoing a left hemispherectomy at the age of two and a half and tested as virtually normal with respect to linguistic ability at age 14, his language faculty now subserved by regions in his right hemisphere (Danelli et al. 2013).

While such instances of plasticity are certainly impressive and reveal that the phenomenon is not confined to sensorimotor cortices alone, more typical examples (indeed, the first to be discovered) involve the expansion of cortical maps to neighboring regions of intact cortex that have been deprived of sensory input from within the same modality as that subserved by the invading cortex, such as might occur when the cortical area corresponding to one manual digit invades the neighboring area corresponding to the adjacent digit following a loss of input to the adjacent digit (Rauschecker 2001). This phenomenon is known as "intramodal" plasticity. The earliest studies of neuroplasticity reported intramodal effects in adult monkeys. Using the topographically arranged somatosensory cortical map as the dependent variable, it was found that when deprived of input, either by median nerve transection or digital amputation, though initially unresponsive, the somatosensory map did not remain unresponsive and was soon activated in response to adjacent inputs (22 days in the case of transection, two to eight months in the case of amputation). Similar results were reported after denervation or amputation in the raccoon, flying fox, cat, and rat, and "large-scale remodeling can occur in human somatosensory and motor cortical areas in the weeks or months immediately following limb amputation" (Buonomano & Merzenich 1998, pp. 163, 165). The results are equally dramatic for the visual and auditory cortices, demonstrating that, "when a given cortical area is deprived of its normal afferent inputs, it reorganizes so that the deprived area becomes responsive to sensory inputs formerly represented only within the cortical sectors surrounding those representing lesioned input sources" (Buonomano & Merzenich 1998, p. 167).

It is as well to note that intramodal plastic changes may be induced without sensory deprivation. Studies on somatosensory, visual, and auditory cortices show that intramodal plastic changes can be induced by training animals on specialized tasks. In humans, magnetoencephalography (MEG) reveals that hand representations of Braille readers are significantly larger for the right index finger than for the left index finger or for the right index finger of non–Braille readers (Pascual-Leone & Torres 1993). Likewise, the digital representation of string players is larger for the left hand than for the right hand or the left hand of control subjects (Elbert et al. 1995).

2.4.2 Crossmodal plasticity

Whereas intramodal plasticity (as its name suggests) occurs *within* a modality, "crossmodal" reorganization involves "expansion of maps in one modality as a result of deprivation in another" (Rauschecker 2001, p. 244). The changes here are more obviously compensatory. Cortical maps used for, say, hearing, might project into occipital cortex following deprivation of visual stimuli, whereupon occipital cortex acquires the processing structures typical of auditory cortex; or visual deprivation might lead to recruitment of primary visual cortex for tactile processing (Noppeney 2007). And since the area supporting the lost function is put to an alternative use, crossmodal plasticity actually makes recovery of the original function quite challenging (Pascual-Leone et al. 2005, p. 395). While it had previously been supposed that interventions must be drastic to induce crossmodal plastic changes, "it is now clear that simply withholding the normal pattern of sensory experience in one modality is sufficient to reorganize the neural representation of the remaining senses"; furthermore, "[i]t appears that the same synaptic mechanisms are invoked that also rule synaptic changes within the same modality" (Rauschecker 2001, pp. 244–245). Crossmodal changes require that cortical maps receive input connections, albeit indirectly, from new epithelial surfaces, and there are essentially two ways for this to occur: either via synaptogenesis, in which new connections are established between the deprived cortical region and a region that already has the relevant connections to the sensory end-organ; or the "unmasking" (strengthening/rearrangement/potentiation) via LTP or some other synaptic plastic mechanism of *existing* connections between the deprived cortex and the sensory end-organ and/or its associated cortex (Rauschecker 2001, p. 255; Ptito, Kupers, et al. 2012). Unmasking is probably preliminary to synaptogenesis (Pascual-Leone et al. 2005, pp. 379, 394–395; Merabet & Pascual-Leone 2010, p. 48). There is experimental support for both mechanisms in crossmodal plasticity, and both are likely to play a role in intramodal plasticity.

The extent of crossmodal plastic change is of course partly a function of time (Noppeney 2007). Short-term changes that enhance the processing capabilities of spared modalities are probably the effects of unmasking and consequently more readily reversible after input restoration (Pascual-Leone et al. 2005, pp. 390–391; Noppeney 2007, p. 1177). Blindfolding induces rapid changes that are just as swiftly reversed after visual input restoration. Long-term deprivation, on the other hand, is more likely to result in sustained structural reorganization through synaptogenesis following initial unmasking (Pascual-Leone et al. 2005, pp. 390–391). This would no doubt explain why the most dramatic crossmodal impacts are observed in cases of early-onset and congenital blindness: "functional reorganization is particularly pronounced in early onset blindness" (Noppeney 2007, p. 1170). The occipital cortices of such subjects, for instance, appear to be functionally important for Braille character identification (although not detection), suggesting a functional contribution of the reorganized occipital cortices in complex tactile discrimination (Noppeney 2007, pp. 1173–1174). Early and congenitally blind subjects routinely outperform sighted subjects in both episodic and semantic memory tasks and may even require the occipital pole for higher-level cognitive and semantic processing (Noppeney 2007, pp. 1171, 1174).

2.4.3 Supramodal (or "metamodal") organization

Not only congenitally and early-blind subjects, but sighted subjects, too, have been found to exhibit occipital cortex activation during nonvisual information processing (Leo et al. 2012, p. 2). The activation in such cases, however, is not straightforwardly crossmodal, since it requires neither sensory deprivation nor special training. While any activation of occipital cortices in sighted subjects performing nonvisual tasks might be ascribed to a preference for *visualizing* nonvisual afferents, the same response pattern in congenitally blind subjects—by definition lacking vision since birth—reveals that some other principle of cortical functional organization is involved. In these cases, occipital cortices do not merely serve as the site for nonvisual information processing, as might be presumed to occur in a standard case of crossmodal plasticity, but seem to be contributing something *visual* to the nonvisual input, and this is no less true for blind subjects (Striem-Amit & Amedi 2014, see p. 21). That is to say, nonvisual information is apparently being processed *visually*, in contrast to crossmodal plasticity, which would (presumably) involve the nonvisual processing of nonvisual afferents, albeit in primary visual cortex. Evidence for the phenomenon, variously termed "supramodal," "metamodal," or "amodal" organization (Pascual-Leone & Hamilton 2001; Striem-Amit & Amedi 2014; Laurence & Margolis 2015), came originally from studies of the dorsal and ventral visual pathways, implicated, respectively, in space and motion discrimination and object/shape-category recognition. More recently, supramodally active regions have been confirmed beyond the occipital cortices (Leo et al. 2012, p. 2).

The nature of supramodal organization is best illustrated by studies involving early and congenitally blind subjects. The dorsal visual pathway of such subjects is active during tactile and auditory motion-discrimination tasks and reflects the activation patterns of sighted controls performing corresponding tasks (Ptito, Matteau et al. 2012, p. 2). Similarly, the ventral visual pathway of early and congenitally blind subjects is active during both haptic (tactile) and nonhaptic (electrotactile) object exploration tasks, again reflecting activations observed in sighted controls performing corresponding tasks (although blind subjects activated larger portions of the ventral stream during nonhaptic tactile shape discrimination than did sighted controls) (Ptito, Matteau et al. 2012, p. 2). In a recent study, it was shown that visual experience in the perception of body shapes is not necessary for the activation of the visual extrastriate body area (EBA) (Striem-Amit & Amedi 2014). Congenitally blind subjects were trained to use a "visual-to-auditory sensory substitution device" that converts visual images into auditory "soundscapes." The EBA was robustly active when subjects were presented with body soundscapes. Hence, "despite the vast plasticity of the cortex to process other sensory inputs" (i.e., crossmodal plasticity), these findings suggest "retention of functional specialization in this same region" (Striem-Amit & Amedi 2014, p. 4). The dorsal and ventral processing streams, and the EBA in particular, appear to be modular, developmentally constrained, and functionally preserved, despite complete early and congenital visual impairment. That they are responsive to sensory information channeled from other modalities also suggests that these regions are not strictly domain-specific, since they are not beholden to specific sensory transduction pathways. Instead, they seem to be sensory-independent and *task*-selective (Striem-Amit & Amedi 2014, p. 5). The preexisting intermodal connections that are unmasked under crossmodal influence may, apparently even in the absence of crossmodal plastic unmasking, supply the critical cortical infrastructure supporting this supramodal dynamic (Pascual-Leone & Hamilton 2001, p. 439; Pascual-Leone et al. 2005, pp. 393–394; Leo et al. 2012, p. 2). The original motivation for domain specificity might have been rationalized in roughly the following way: Any module must (minimally) have a specific function it "knows" to perform on just the right occasion/s. Cognitive scientists can explain this with the suggestion that a specific input or external stimulus cues the module to respond (Pascual-Leone & Hamilton 2001, p. 431). What supramodal organization vividly demonstrates, however, is that inputs need *not* be external stimuli—internally mediated stimuli across modalities are normal—and that any *one* module will typically be sensitive to *more than one* stimulus, including those channeled along intermodal pathways. Put another way, it would appear that modules are frequently *reused*.[4] I shall explain this in greater detail in Chapter 3.

Compelling evidence of supramodal organization also comes from subjects whose senses are intact. (This material does not address the kind of plasticity we have been considering so far in this chapter, but it is related in ways that will become clearer in Chapter 3, as well as Chapter 6.) It had already been known that unisensory cortices may be active when presented with stimuli coming through other modalities, as when a single stimulus component of a typically bimodal event with a close semantic connection is presented on its own; for example the sound of tools, the voice of a loved one, the sight of lips mouthing words, and such like (Hirst et al. 2012). Learning and conditioning of arbitrary pairings of unrelated stimuli may also produce these results (Hirst et al. 2012, p. 2). What was not confirmed until recently is whether these results depended on a prior semantic association, or otherwise "an explicit conditioning paradigm, or prolonged, habitual co-occurrence of bimodal stimuli" (Hirst et al. 2012, p. 2). Hirst et al.'s (2012) clinical study confirmed that, even without sensory deficits, training, or semantic associations, primary visual cortex exhibits an increased number of active neurons when presented with sounds alone, provided that subjects are pre-exposed to the auditory and visual stimuli. There is also evidence that the occipital cortex of sighted subjects is active during tactile processing of orientation, and, perhaps most astonishingly, that semantic word-generation in sighted subjects depends partly on bilateral occipital cortices, regions that have always been supposed to be among the most specialized in the brain (Pascual-Leone et al. 2005, p. 394). Studies by Antonio Damasio and Alex Martin were among the first to demonstrate activation of motor areas during

---

[4] Cf. Barrett & Kurzban (2006, pp. 634–635), who argue that something like task selectivity defines *formal* domain specificity, although it is often enough construed as evidence of a domain-general system: they observe that "there is no natural line that separates domain-specific from domain-general mechanisms." See my § 5.1 for elaboration.

verb-retrieval tasks and visual areas during noun-processing tasks, such as naming colors and animals (Damasio & Tranel 1993; Damasio et al. 1996; Martin et al. 1995, 1996, 2000). Merely the sight of manipulatable artifacts—indeed, just seeing their names—activates parts of the brain associated with prehension (Chao & Martin 2000).

The material presented in this chapter is by no means intended to serve as an exhaustive or even necessarily comprehensive account of the fascinating field of neuroplasticity. But what I have provided ought to be sufficient to support the claims I make in Chapter 6. In the next chapter, I provide a synopsis of what could well be regarded as yet another class of neuroplastic responses: responses that are, however, sufficiently distinctive in character when compared with cortical map plasticity and memory consolidation as to warrant separate consideration.

2.5 Summary

The brain exhibits an impressive degree of plasticity. Plasticity is really an intrinsic feature of the nervous system, not an exceptional or occasional state. Neuroplasticity comprises a family of different types of plasticity. Of these, synaptic plasticity is perhaps the best-understood variety and plays an important role in cortical map reorganization and memory consolidation. Cortical map plasticity is of direct relevance to any discussion of modularity. There are two types of cortical map plasticity: intramodal and crossmodal. Crossmodal plasticity is likely to arise from the underlying supramodal (or "metamodal") organization of the brain.

3

Neural Reuse and Recycling

3.1 What is Neural Reuse?

Our brief survey of neuroplasticity led us to a consideration of one rather striking feature of neural organization: what is variously termed "supramodal," "metamodal," or "amodal" organization. This feature of brain organization makes it possible for a region of the brain typically responsive to a unique stimulus to respond to input mediated by a different modality, and thus enable the cooperation of neural ensembles in the absence of standard inputs. We saw that supramodal plastic changes may be distinguished from crossmodal changes by virtue of the altered regions' retaining something of their original character and neural function—their contribution has not been wholly, or in many cases even primarily, subordinated to the processing demands of the alternative modality. That such ensembles appear to be operative in normally sighted and hearing adult subjects suggests, furthermore—perhaps somewhat surprisingly—that supramodal organization is a latent feature of the normally functioning brain. We must now stop to consider how such evidence forces us to rethink some basic assumptions in cognitive and neural science. It is not the recruitment of multiple brain areas or modules that gives pause for thought here, for no doubt complex tasks will require a degree of intermodular cooperation. What is striking is the possibility of significantly more overlaps between the neural regions implicated in higher cognitive functions than the standard picture allows, and hence the sharing of neural resources at a much finer level of detail (i.e., in a vastly more promiscuous fashion) than previously acknowledged. Taken overall, the evidence rather suggests that what we might initially *think* of as basic modular units could resolve into still more basic domain-general (i.e., task-selective) elements, and that hitherto grossly specified functions such as vision and language cannot be located in functionally dedicated regions of the brain. The evidence is thus compatible with the deep interpenetration of higher level psychological functions, as distinct from merely their co-option.

The Adaptable Mind. John Zerilli, Oxford University Press (2021). © Oxford University Press.
DOI: 10.1093/oso/9780190067885.003.0003

One of the core principles of neuroscience is the principle of functional localization, the idea that specific brain functions "can be mapped to local structure in a relatively straightforward way" (Anderson 2010, p. 245; Gold & Roskies 2008, p. 354). Modern neuroscience is largely predicated on the discovery of such structures and reckons success when a relatively discrete anatomical site can be correlated with some aspect of behavior or function. Still, it has never been entirely clear to what extent, or in just what way, this assumption can be justified. For one thing, some obvious questions immediately obtrude: "The main questions to be answered by any theory that claims that the mind consists of parts are *Which* parts? and Why *those* parts?" (Ohlsson 1994, p. 724). Holding that mental functions fall along such axes as language, mathematics, physics, psychology, and so on, calls for a principled defense of this selection, but at times the choice seems a trite folksy, not to say arbitrary. Behind these questions lies the more specific issue of how any supposed carve-up might square with psychological data demonstrating the apparently interactive structure of many behaviors, even those as simple as reflexes (Amaral & Strick 2013, p. 337). How is a fact like supramodal organization, by virtue of which bilateral occipital cortices appear to be standardly redeployed in semantic language tasks, to be accounted for on the assumption that brain areas are highly specialized? At least one thing is abundantly clear: "functional differences . . . cannot be accounted for primarily by differences in which brain regions get utilized—as they are reused across domains" (Anderson 2010, p. 247).

Evidence of the "reuse," "recycling," or "redeployment" of brain areas is now extensive (Dehaene 2005; Anderson 2007a, 2007b, 2007c, 2008, 2010, 2014). These terms refer to the "exaptation" of established and relatively fixed neural circuits over the course of evolution or normal development, generally without loss of original function.[1] "[R]ather than posit a functional architecture for the brain whereby individual regions are dedicated to large-scale cognitive domains like vision, audition, language and the like, neural reuse theories suggest that low-level neural circuits are used and reused for various purposes in different cognitive and task domains" (Anderson 2010, p. 246). Speaking of an increasingly familiar example of the reuse of an area once thought to be highly specialized, the neurolinguist David Poeppel remarks:

---

[1] This usage of "exaptation" is somewhat misleading, since exaptation usually implies loss of original function (see Godfrey-Smith 2001).

A statement such as "Broca's area underpins language production" (or "speech," or "syntax," or other broad categories of linguistic experience) is not just grossly underspecified, it is ultimately both misleading and incorrect. Broca's region is not monolithic but instead is comprised of numerous subregions as specified by cytoarchitecture, immunocytochemistry, laminar properties, and so on. And domains of language such as "syntax" are similarly not monolithic but shorthand for complex suites of underlying representations and computations. It is perhaps not surprising that a brain area such as Broca's region is therefore implicated in many functions, some of which are not even particularly tied to language. . . . Future work ought to focus on "decomposing" or fractionating such complex psychological functions into putative primitive operations to account for the wide range of phenomena that are mediated by anatomically complex brain structures such as Broca's area. (2015, p. 140)

Language coarsely characterized as a gross function (or subfunction; e.g., recursion) appears to disarticulate into much finer functional granules whose computational resources are available both within and outside the domain of language. This is the essence of the theory of reuse: it explains overlapping neural activation with the suggestion that far smaller functional units with structured operations are used and reused across various task categories. Perhaps many statements that have now attained the status of platitudes— such as "Lining up objects does not form the basis of word order. Trying to fit one toy inside another has nothing to do with embedded clauses" (Karmiloff-Smith 1994, p. 698)—have in fact been premature. In what follows here and the next few chapters, I shall certainly argue that this is so, inspired as I am by a commitment to the basic principle that intuitions about cognitive functions need always to be examined (and reexamined) in the light of what neuroscience actually reveals, even where this looks to be at odds with what comparative psychology or linguistics suggests about uniquely human, uniquely linguistic cognitive feats (see, e.g., Chomsky 1965, pp. 58–59). The comparative psychologist might well ask: "If word order is just object discrimination and sequencing, and recursion some sort of applied folk physics, why is it that chimpanzees have nothing even approaching a human language system, though they manifest rich sensorimotor and representational abilities?" There is no shame in confessing that the answer here is by no means clear, which is no doubt why many continue to hold out hope that at the very least *some* aspects of language processing might not just be uniquely human, but also uniquely linguistic. One dares suggest that there might well be a small or even exiguous component of otherwise highly interpenetrated circuits that is rarely reused outside the language domain, and that would in consequence be specialized in a strict sense—a mechanism recruited for linguistic purposes and little else, dedicated by virtue not only of its isolable functional contribution and circumscribed circuitry, but also its dedication to a specific task category. Consider the possibility of a neuron or tightly restricted set of neurons being dedicated to, say, conjugating the verb "to be" and having no nonlinguistic functions at all (Prinz 2006). This component might aptly be described as a language "module" (or "minimodule") for all practical purposes (see Chapter 4), and I shall consider its prospects in Chapter 7.

For the present, it suffices to remark that the evidence to which Poeppel refers in the extract cited earlier cannot be ignored either. The fusiform gyrus was rather wistfully hailed as the "face area" after the discovery that it responds to human faces suggested it could be a special-purpose device (Kanwisher et al. 1997). It was later found that the area responds to other categories of objects for which it appears we have expertise, such as cars, birds, and traveling objects (Gauthier et al. 2000). Even the more fundamental notion that ventral visual processing areas are specialized for shape discrimination has been called into question by evidence that information about many objects is distributed across the cortex, and that in some cases their identities can be recovered from low-level activation patterns across several occipital cortices (Haxby et al. 2001; Hanson et al. 2004). I detail further evidence of neural reuse in § 3.3. For the moment, we must turn to consider what is arguably the leading theoretical exposition of reuse attracting serious attention in cognitive science, neuroscience, and philosophy: Michael Anderson's massive redeployment hypothesis.

3.2 The Massive Redeployment Hypothesis

Neural reuse theories comprise what Anderson describes as "an emerging class of theories," which, "taken together . . . offer a new research-guiding idealization of brain organization" (Anderson 2010, p. 246). Anderson's own hypothesis builds on the assumption that *evolution* might prefer the reuse of neural circuitry over the development of new circuitry *de novo* (Anderson 2010, p. 246). From this assumption, three predictions are thought to follow, the most obvious being neural reuse itself. "A typical brain region [should] support numerous cognitive functions in diverse task categories." Second, older brain areas should, *ceteris paribus*, be reused more than newer ones, because "having been available for reuse for longer," they are likelier candidates for integration into recently evolved functions.[2] Third, recently evolved functions should be more distributed than older ones since it should on the whole prove easier to utilize available circuits than to devise special-purpose circuitry afresh, "and there is little reason to suppose that the useful elements will happen to reside in neighboring brain regions." Conversely, "a more localist account of the evolution of the brain would . . . expect the continual development of new, largely dedicated neural circuits" for every cognitive innovation or significant increase in cognitive power.

Anderson has tested these predictions in a number of studies, with conspicuous success (2007a; 2007c; 2008). For instance, the typical cortical region was found to be implicated in fully nine domains extending from action, vision, and audition through language, mathematics, memory, and reasoning. This illustrates an important feature of reuse; that is, the possibility (in principle) of congruously overlapping regions—just the same circuits exapted for one purpose can be exapted for another, provided sufficient intercircuit pathways exist to allow alternative arrangements of them. The same parts put together in different ways will yield different functional outcomes, just as "if one puts together the same parts *in the same way* one will get the same functional outcomes" (Anderson 2010, p. 247, my emphasis) (see Fig. 3.1).

Regarding the second prediction, that older areas are more likely to be reused than recently evolved regions, if we make the simplifying assumption that older areas lie at the back of the brain, Anderson's results confirm the expectation. Anderson reports a negative correlation between the position of a brain region along the Y-axis in Tailarach space[3] and the number of tasks that activate the region. The results were replicated using different data sets, with Anderson evaluating them in this vein:

Although the amount of variance explained in these cases is not especially high, the findings are nevertheless striking, at least in part because a more

---

[2] The evolutionary psychologist's invocation of so-called debugging concerns is addressed in § 5.1.

[3] "Tailarach space" is the three-dimensional human brain atlas used by neuroscientists for mapping locations in brain space—the correlation is counterintuitively reported as "negative" because in Tailarach space, the origin is set at the center of the brain, with regions posterior measured in negative coordinates.

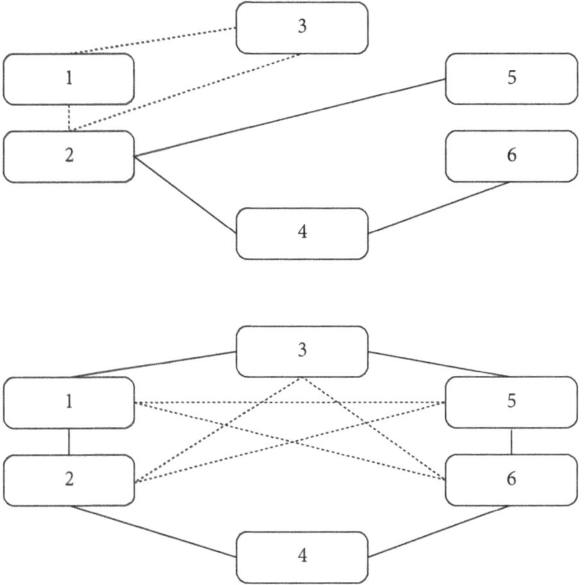

Figure 3.1 Two cognitive functions indicated by solid and dashed lines, organized in the top figure the way that an anatomical account of modularity would predict, and in the bottom figure in accordance with how neural reuse sees the matter. Anatomical modularity maintains functional dissociability and localization for gross or high-level functions with few if any overlapping units. Reuse suggests overlapping units that form different patterns of connection.

(Michael L. Anderson, "Neural reuse: A fundamental organizational principle of the brain," *Behavioral and Brain Sciences*, Volume 33, Issue 4, August 2010, pp. 245–266. Reproduced with permission of Cambridge University Press.)

traditional theory of functional topography would predict the *opposite* re-lation, if there were any relation at all. According to traditional theories, older areas—especially those visual areas at the back of the brain—are ex-pected to be the *most* domain dedicated. But that is not what the results show. (2010, p. 247)

As for the third prediction, that recently evolved functions ought to gen-erate more distributed patterns of activation than older ones, Anderson's (2007a) findings suggest that language could well be the paradigm, supported by more distributed activations than visual perception and attention, and in-deed than any other domain that was tested (Anderson 2008). Results such as these showing widely scattered activations across the brain for putatively late-developing functions are incidentally consistent with the degree of specialization for local circuits that neural reuse actually presupposes. For neural reuse *is* of course consistent with a certain kind of specialization: as the very word "redeployment" suggests, it presupposes the existence of comparatively fixed neural circuits whose functional contribution may be preserved across multiple task domains. The metabolic costs of maintaining long-distance connections would presumably encourage the reuse of local flexible ("polyfunctional") circuits, if any were around; "[t]hat this is not the observed pattern suggests that some functionally relevant aspect of local circuits is relatively fixed" (Anderson 2010, p. 247; but cf. Anderson 2014, pp. 15–16, 104).[4] Anderson's earliest formulations of the redeployment hypothesis accounted for this fixity by introducing an important distinction, following Bergeron (2007, 2008), between stable, low-level computational "workings" (or cortical "biases") and diverse higher level cognitive "uses." Workings are represented in the numbered units of Fig. 3.1, while uses are represented by the functional composites formed from these units. Workings are really very tiny regions of cortex that make a specific computational contribution to higher-level cognitive tasks or "uses." We might say that workings represent an essential functional contribution across all task categories, considered in isolation of neural context (although Anderson has since moved away from essentialism), and that uses are the higher level cognitive functions enabled by the composite of several workings. (More on this in Chapter 4.)

Stable structure for local circuits is a feature of a closely related account of neural reuse, one that posits reuse or recycling as a *developmental* solution (in contrast to Anderson, for whom reuse was, originally, primarily an evolutionary solution). How are readily transmissible cultural practices whose phylogenetic emergence is too recent for evolutionary hardwiring to explain, such as reading and arithmetic, to be neurophysiologically accounted for? Early developmental neuroplasticity might be one way, but in supposing that local circuits might be too rigid for the effects of experience to overcome, Dehaene (2005) gives priority to "neuronal recycling."

Of course, neuroplasticity is not something either Dehaene or Anderson would wish to deny. Dehaene goes as far as accepting (as I think one must) that novel uses that depart significantly from existing cortical biases cannot simply be exapted from them: a high-level use that places a significant

---

[4] Scattered activations can be explained other than by the suggestion that local circuits are relatively fixed. I return to this issue in Chapter 5 (see § 5.1).

cognitive burden on existing circuits, themselves better suited for other uses, must in the end disrupt those circuits and the alternative uses to which they might be put. More cognitively demanding functional acquisitions therefore require more neuroplasticity. This brings us to a potentially thorny issue. Just what is the relationship between reuse and plasticity? There might seem to be a tension between the fixity necessary to get reuse off the ground on one hand, and the plasticity necessary for reuse to play an interesting role in learning and evolutionary novelty on the other. In fact there is no real problem here (Anderson & Finlay 2014). Anderson describes neural reuse as a change in use without a change in working, and plasticity as a change in use resulting *from* a change in working (Anderson 2010, p. 297). There is no real problem here because some forms of neuroplasticity (such as Hebbian synaptic plasticity) do not *require* flexible units before they can effect a change in use, given that they involve only adjustments to connection strength ("a change in use without a change in working"); besides that, neural units are not quite so "fixed" as Anderson's own (2010) remarks suggest, allowing for more drastic forms of neuroplasticity (such as synaptogenesis and the like) to partly override the natural biases of particular brain regions ("a change in use from a change in working"). I will revisit these themes in Chapter 6 (see p. 93).

It might be just as well to point out one other respect in which the story of neural reuse is compatible with the known biophysical constraints and possibilities of neural circuits. Neural reuse is really an ideal solution to what might be called the *scaling problem* (Zador 2015, p. 43; Bullmore & Sporns 2012, pp. 337–339). "The scaling problem" refers to the dilemma that, as the number of neurons increases, undoubtedly conferring advantages in the form of increased behavioral flexibility and intelligence, the number of neurons that must be connected before such advantages can materialize grows quadratically larger. Thus, in a small 10-neuron circuit, only 100 connections are required, but in a larger circuit consisting of perhaps 100 million neurons, anywhere up to a thousand billion connections might be required. It is not easy to see, from the point of view of engineering and design, how an ever larger brain can be wired up efficiently when the number of neural connections required soon becomes immense. This consideration has actually been played as an argument in favor of modularity, but it could just as well be pressed into the service of neural reuse, which delivers fixed low-level cognitive workings that operate autonomously in something like the way of traditional modules (see § 5.1).

3.3 Further Evidence of Neural Reuse

3.3.1 Computational modeling

A number of large-scale computational models of the brain are currently being developed in the hope of understanding the activity of a million neurons or more. At their most sophisticated, they leave behind the biologically unrealistic neural network models of the past and enter the domain of real brain simulation, neurorobotics, and neuromorphic computing. As the computational analogues of real neural networks, they are beginning to offer fresh insights into the brain's dynamic response properties. The primary advantage of brain simulation is that, "unlike the empirical brain, the model's internal workings are completely known and the model's structure can be modified in order to explore how its activity changes" (Sporns 2015, p. 97). One example of brain simulation that is especially relevant in the present context is SPAUN (Semantic Pointer Architecture Unified Network). Spaun has a single eye through which it receives digital images as input, and a moving arm through which it provides behavioral output (Eliasmith 2015). What is interesting is that its 2.5 million "neurons" are organized to simulate about twenty of the roughly one thousand functionally distinct areas that neuroscientists typically identify in the brain (e.g., separate neurons for frontal cortex, basal ganglia, occipital cortex, etc.). One feature of Spaun that supports the theory of reuse comes as a result of this unique "modular" architecture:

> One key contribution of Spaun relative to many competing architectures is that Spaun can perform a variety of different behaviours, much like an actual brain. For example, Spaun can use its visual system to recognize numbers that it then organizes into a list and then stores in working memory. It can then later recall this list and draw the numbers, in order, using its arm. Furthermore, Spaun can use this same visual system to parse more complex input. . . . To do so, it uses the same memory system, but in a slightly different way. As well, it uses other brain areas that it didn't use in the list recall task. *That is, Spaun can deploy the same brain areas in different ways depending on what task it needs to perform.* (Eliasmith 2015, p. 132, my emphasis)

Spaun's differentiated circuits manifest the very same interactive dynamics that reuse posits of real brains: "different, specialized brain areas are *coordinated* in a task-specific—that is, *flexible*—way to meet a challenge presented by the environment" (Eliasmith 2015, p. 132). This behavioral flexibility marks a distinctive sense in which neural reuse is a form of plasticity: the ability to switch effortlessly from task to task (reading an email, playing a piano, chasing a dog) using the same brain areas in different ways and with little or no delay in shuffling between them. This kind of plasticity serves to set biological intelligence apart from most contemporary artificial intelligence, and indeed explains why Spaun is "atypical of the field" overall (Eliasmith 2015, p. 134). Most machines are good at doing one specific thing (playing chess, solving mathematical equations, driving a car, etc.). Spaun is unique both in the variety of tasks it can perform and its capacity to learn new behaviors independently "while preserving abilities it already has" (Eliasmith 2015, p. 134). Spaun may be one of the first tentative steps towards showing that a domain-general learning system can work.[5]

3.3.2 Biobehavioral evidence

Casasanto and Dijkstra (2010) report an interesting association between autobiographical memory and motor control. The task involved shifting marbles upward or downward from one container to another while relating memories having either positive or negative valence. Subjects were asked to retell, for example, a negative memory, followed by another negative memory, then perhaps a positive memory, while simultaneously moving marbles from one container to another in a given direction. It was found that subjects retrieved more memories, and moved the marbles more quickly, when the direction of movement aligned with the valance of the memory; i.e., when the upward movement coincided with positive memories, and the downward movement with negative memories. Even when subjects were not asked to relate memories that were specifically positive or negative, but just to relate memories as they came, they were more likely to retrieve memories whose valence correlated with the direction of movement. The directedness of the movements involved suggests an important association between

---

[5] Google scientists have pulled off something similar with Agent (Mnih et al. 2015).

memory, movement, and spatial orientation likely to be reflected in shared neural circuitry.

The reuse of spatio-visual circuits for numerical cognition is illustrated by the spatial-numerical association of response codes (SNARC) effect. Here are just two examples of the SNARC effect (Dehaene et al. 1993): (i) when asked whether a number is even or odd, subjects respond more quickly with large numbers displayed to their right, or small numbers to their left; (ii) when presented with a line of neutral symbols (e.g., XXXXX) subjects fare better at correctly indicating the midpoint than when presented with small numbers (e.g., 22222), in which case there is a bias to the left, or large numbers (e.g., 99999), where the bias is to the right. It appears that in these cases a mental number line running from left to right is being navigated with the help of spatial orientation circuits (Hubbard et al. 2005).

3.3.3 Final thoughts

Despite the extensive and compelling nature of the evidence supporting reuse, not to mention again the powerful evolutionary considerations in its favor, the case has not yet managed to convince everyone. Neural activation and imaging evidence on its own is ambiguous, the skeptics point out, being consistent with multiple neighboring sets of neurons that only *appear* to be reused as a result of the coarse spatial resolution of contemporary imaging technologies (Anderson 2010, pp. 298–299; 2014, p. 29). Furthermore,

> . . . because neural activation may spread around the brain network, this can lead to false positives: regions that are activated only as a side effect of their connectivity and not because they are making a functional contribution to the task under investigation. (Anderson 2014, p. 29)

This "spreading activation" is what Colin Klein (2010, p. 280) has dubbed a "potential confound," and such worries cannot be lightly dismissed. On the contrary, misgivings about the use of neuroimaging evidence are precisely why converging biobehavioral evidence (of the kind just cited) will be critical in a debate like this. The more biobehavioral evidence of functional and semantic inheritance between task domains, the greater our confidence that the very same neural structures are involved (Anderson 2014, p. 30). The limitations of neuroimaging technology can thus be overcome by adopting supplementary research paradigms. An interference paradigm, for example, asks participants to process two stimuli at the same time. If the processing of these stimuli draws on shared neural resources, one would expect this to be reflected in performance: perhaps a slower reaction time as compared to performance on similar tasks that do not make processing demands on the same neural elements. Thus, on the assumption that the fusiform face area would respond to objects of expertise as well as faces, Gauthier et al. (2003) predicted that face processing in car experts would be impeded by the presentation of cars at the same time—and this is just what they found. Here we have evidence of reuse coming from a research paradigm outside neuroimaging, and none the worse for that. Later on I cite yet a further type of evidence, this time from single-neuron studies, demonstrating that, while concerns over poor spatial resolution and spreading activation may be legitimate, they can hardly be decisive (see the discussion of "strong context effects" in § 5.1). The simple fact of the matter is that evidence in support of reuse comes from many quarters, including from disciplines—such as neurology and neuropsychology—in which distributed parallel processing models had been proposed well *before* the advent of neuroimaging technology (Bressler 1995, p. 289). Still, even assuming that the general thrust of this hypothesis is correct (as I for one do), it is not immediately obvious that anatomical modularity is dead, for perhaps it is only in respect of its functional scope that it stands in need of revision. Moreover, as I suggested earlier in this chapter, outstanding questions concerning the existence of a dedicated language module remain as acute as ever, and these are tied in part to an extensive dissociation literature as well as to the concerns over spatial resolution and neuroimaging I just raised. I turn now to consider these issues, and begin by inquiring into just what the implications of reuse and neuroplasticity might be for the modularity of mind.

3.4 Summary

"Neural reuse" refers to the exaptation of established and relatively fixed neural circuits without loss of original function/use. Reuse arises over the course of normal development and evolution. The evidence of this phenomenon speaks most loudly against the idea of strict domain-specificity. It seems that no area of the brain is exempt from redeployment, with areas of the brain traditionally considered to be among the most domain-specific (such as sensory areas) also contributing their computational/structural resources to other domains, including those involving language. The evidence supporting reuse takes many forms, among them evolutionary and developmental considerations, computational considerations, and the neuroimaging and biobehavioral literature.

4

Modules Reconsidered

Varieties of Modularity

4.1 A Pivot to the Neurosciences

Evidence of neural reuse points to an overall picture of the brain that has disruptive implications for the modularity of mind, particularly for classical varieties of the theory such as Fodor's, massive modularity, and Adaptive Control of Thought—Rational (ACT-R), which all posit modules for high-level cognitive functions or proprietary domains. No doubt many will resist this assessment. I certainly have sympathy for the tradition of functional decomposition and shall not in any case be recommending that we dispense with modules here. Nonetheless, such evidence of reuse as we have clearly does point to "the need for a supplement to business as usual" (Anderson 2010, p. 249).

The central problem for modularity, at least as it has traditionally been understood, is that modules talk lends itself most naturally to the analogy of bricks and mortar, or the assembly of component parts. As an intricately dense network of synaptic connections, electrical signals, and neuromodulatory dynamics, however, the brain is nowhere obviously organized in this bricks and mortar sort of way, even where it sometimes proves fruitful to account for neurobiological function in mechanistic compositional terms (Craver 2007; Bechtel 2008b). The question is whether the bricks and mortar analogy is so far superseded by the network analogy that there is no longer any residual value in speaking of modules at all. If the brain is not obviously or even predominantly an assembly of functional components, surely it would not be unreasonable to hope that any theory having as its target the mind's functional organization would adequately accommodate itself to this fact.

The brain's network structure notwithstanding, metaphors, it seems, die hard, especially ones freighted with as much philosophical baggage as modularity. It may be that metaphors are all we have, but if so, we are going to need the right ones. To those reluctant to give up on the modular perspective,

The Adaptable Mind. John Zerilli, Oxford University Press (2021). © Oxford University Press.
DOI: 10.1093/oso/9780190067885.003.0004

I hope my own recommendation of a substantial yet cautious reform may offer some consolation. My proposal is simple—that we recalibrate our notion of modules in deference to what currently passes for a module in contemporary mainstream neuroscience. Cognitive scientists and philosophers whose work is attentive to the neurosciences already think in these terms, and it is not hard to appreciate why: when it comes to modularity, which concerns the functional *organization* of the mind, psychological theorizing is even more constrained by issues of implementation than might generally be the case. For some reason, however, many philosophers continue to talk about modules in a manner conveying either ignorance of what neuroscience has to say about the structure of the brain, or else a breezy indifference. A reorientation towards neuroscience entails a shift of focus away from understanding modules as unimodal higher level cognitive mechanisms and towards a conception of modules as metamodal (i.e., reusable) nodes subserving exiguous low-level subfunctions. I argue that a module built on this pattern, sometimes called a "brain module," can serve as an appropriate revisionary benchmark for cognitive scientists and philosophers of psychology still wedded to the idea of classical modules. Notice, however, that this proposal also entails a certain agnosticism regarding the prospects of modularity in the long run. Being sensitive to developments in the neurosciences means being willing to part with long-cherished notions if need be. It so happens that further evidence of neural reuse presented in the next chapter may necessitate a profounder shift away from traditional modules than the one I am currently recommending. Hence I am urging a recalibration in the face of developments that will either, if all goes well, allow us to safeguard a respectable (though revised) notion of modularity, or, should things not turn out so well, undermine its rationale comprehensively—this is where the real battle lines are being drawn. Later on I shall suggest one way that we might usefully conceptualize the issues presented by these developments. Still, the broader point remains: if modules exist at all—a question on which it pays not to be dogmatic one way or the other—they will not resemble the modules of classical cognitive science.

In the next section, I provide a rough sketch of the varieties of modularity one might expect to come across in the cognitive sciences. In this section I also defend what I take to be the *sine qua non* of modularity; namely, functional dissociability. This will be important in heading off an obvious objection to the argument I am making here: that modules can always survive *qua* abstract, higher level/gross functional "systems." I follow this section with a basic account of the brain module. The next chapter pursues at greater length the central question of this book—Whither modularity?—in the hope of demonstrating why neural reuse points us in the direction of something like the brain module.

4.2 Varieties of Modularity

4.2.1 Themes and trends

The nineteenth-century phrenologists were probably the first to emphasize the specialization of brain functions. Gall and Spurzheim (1835) hypothesized that there were "about thirty-five affective and intellectual faculties" localized in distinct regions of the brain. As almost everyone knows, however, they got the details horribly wrong, for they fallaciously assumed that the activity of a cortical faculty would be reflected in its size, and that its size in turn would be reflected in the relative prominence of cranial bumps. This led them to endorse the pseudoscientific practice of gauging personality from the shape of a person's skull. Wrong though they most assuredly were in this respect, the idea that brain function can be mapped to local structure was not itself a bad idea. It soon received empirical support in the work of the neurologists Gustav Fritsch, Eduard Hitzig, Paul Broca, and Carl Wernicke—Broca and Wernicke being of course the first to discover the so-called "language areas" of the brain (Bridgeman 2010). Indeed, by the end of the nineteenth century, the idea of mapping the brain was well on its way to becoming the equipment of every working scientist in the field. In fact "the notion of cognitive function being subdivided and routed to different regions of the brain has remained a central idea in neural science and a fundamental principle in the clinical practice of neurology" (Pascual-Leone & Hamilton 2001, p. 431).

Corresponding to a rough division between "mind" and "brain," one may trace the course of two distinct but parallel traditions originating in the work of these nineteenth-century neurologists. The first is a *structuralist* tradition whose methodology, guiding assumptions, and theoretical concerns are predominantly biological (i.e., neurological and anatomical). From a certain point of view, Fodor's archetype could be said to fall broadly within this tradition—notwithstanding the subordinate and strictly dispensable role played by structural properties in his overall account (Anderson &

Finlay 2014, p. 5; Fodor 1983, pp. 71, 98–99; Coltheart 1999)—as may both the neural network graph-theoretic module (see § 4.2.2) and neuroscience "brain module" (see § 4.3), which I come to shortly.

An alternative approach investigates questions of cognitive architecture from the standpoint of a classic computationalist or functionalist. In the guise of evolutionary psychology or "massive modularity," for example, it "retains the Fodorian focus on *computation*, and with it a focus on the algorithmic (or heuristic) efficiency of purported psychological solutions to adaptive problems such as food choice, mate selection, kin identification and cheater detection" (Anderson & Finlay 2014, p. 5). It does not, however, entail specific commitments about implementation beyond those required for functional independence.[1] (See Sternberg 2011, pp. 158–159, for an overview.)

These two (ideally) complementary approaches to the mind/brain are reflected again in the central assumptions underpinning much of the effort within neuropsychology, cognitive neuropsychology, and cognitive neuroscience (Bergeron 2007). Bergeron calls these the "anatomical modularity assumption" and the "functional modularity assumption." Recall that in Chapter 1, we provided a general definition of an anatomical module. It is worthwhile restating this definition in such a way as to reveal more clearly its relationship to a "functional" module. The functional modularity assumption

> is the idea that the architecture of human cognition largely consists in a configuration of cognitive modules, where a "module" is roughly defined, following Jerry Fodor (1983), as a domain specific, innately specified, and informationally encapsulated system. . . . What this means is that human cognition can be decomposed into a number of functionally independent processes, and that each of these processes operates over a distinct domain of cognitive information. Moreover, since these processes are brain processes, to hypothesize that the capacity to do A and B depends on two distinct cognitive modules—one responsible for the capacity to do A and the other responsible for the capacity to do B—is to hypothesize that the brain processes cognitive information related to A separately from the way it processes cognitive information related to B. . . .

---

[1] Defenders of massive modularity also part company with Fodor's "central"/"peripheral" distinction. Fodor's hypothesis is that only peripheral systems are likely to be modular "to some interesting extent" (1983, p. 37); i.e., sensory input and motor systems. Proponents of massive modularity think that the central systems will be modular, too; i.e., those involved in higher perceptual function, belief-fixation, and inferential reasoning (Sperber 1994, 2002; Carruthers 2006; see also Barrett & Kurzban 2006 and Prinz 2006 for reviews). See my § 7.2.2.

> What makes the A module/process distinct from the B module/process is their *functional independence*, the fact that one can be affected, *in part or in totality*, without the other being affected, and *vice versa*. (Bergeron 2007, pp. 175–176)

The anatomical modularity assumption, then,

> is the idea that the cognitive modules which compose cognition (or at least most of them) each reside in some specific and relatively small portion of the brain. . . . *The anatomical modularity assumption is in fact the functional modularity assumption plus a claim about the implementation of functionally modular processes in the brain.* (Bergeron 2007, p. 176, my emphasis)

Stripped to their essentials, functional modularity implies functional dissociability, while anatomical modularity implies *both* functional dissociability *and* neural localization. As I argue later, functional dissociability—functional modularity, pure and simple—represents the essence of any modular account worthy of the name.

What I have so far failed to mention, though it will in fact be crucial to appreciating the implications of neural reuse, is that cognitive modules have been generally postulated to account for *higher level* or *gross* cognitive functions; i.e., for the sorts of psychological capacities that might appear in the ontologies of cognitive psychology. Even if one restricts one's gaze to the history of the structuralist/neurological tradition, one will not be surprised to learn that, in the main, the project of mapping function to structure has proceeded with a fairly coarse taxonomy of psychological capacities in hand. The phrenologists, for their part, merely translated the categories of Thomas Reid's faculty psychology onto a plan of the skull (acquisitiveness, friendship, sagacity, cautiousness, veneration, etc.) (Poldrack 2010, p. 753). Broca's postulation of a "language" area associated with motor aphasia, though no doubt empirically better supported than Gall and Spurzheim's assumptions, hardly served to sharpen the focus on what the brain itself is actually doing when facilitating speech; for "what warrants the thought that [such] characteristics [as those found in faculty psychology] will be useful to structuring the neuroscience of behaviour and divide the brain at its functional joints?" (Anderson 2014, p. xvi). Consider Russell Poldrack's illuminating *reductio ad absurdum* (cited in Anderson 2014):

> Imagine that fMRI [*functional magnetic resonance imaging*] had been invented in the late 1860s rather than the 1990s. Instead of being based on modern cognitive psychology, neuroimaging would instead be based on the faculty psychology of Thomas Reid and Dugald Steward, which provided the mental "faculties" that Gall and the phrenologists attempted to map onto the brain. Researchers would . . . almost certainly have found brain regions that were reliably engaged when a particular faculty was engaged, . . . [and] Gall and his contemporaries would have taken those neuroimaging results as evidence for the biological reality of his proposed faculties. (Poldrack 2010, p. 753)

What reasons have we for imagining that the taxonomies of modern day psychology will fare any better in carving the brain at its true functional joints? Clinical evidence of dissociations aside (about which I shall have more to say later), widespread evidence of neural reuse strongly suggests that attempts that seek to impose upon the brain a set of categories devised (largely) autonomously of the brain, and molded from a wholly different set of considerations from those guiding brain science generally, are doomed to repeat the same basic phrenological mistake. What is needed is "the development of ontologies that let the phenomena speak on something closer to their own terms" (Anderson 2014, p. xvii).

The structuralist tradition in fact does admit of some exceptions to this questionable trend in what might even be seen by some as a clear premonition of neural reuse theories. As Bergeron's (2007) helpful discussion reminds us, the fact that Carl Wernicke postulated a sensory speech area, often wrongly dubbed the "language comprehension area," makes it all too easy to forget that Wernicke himself was "very resistant to postulating any cerebral centers beyond what he referred to as the 'primary' (motor and perceptual) 'psychic functions'" (2007, p. 184). Wernicke could well be credited with the elaboration of an entirely original approach to the structure–function relationship in the brain. In this approach, only the sensory and motor functions are allocated distinct and dedicated neural anatomy. Higher psychological functions such as those implicated in language production and comprehension are supposed to depend on the interactions of these low-level sensory-motor systems. This arguably anticipates modern theories of reuse that predict that higher cognitive functions resolve in the interactions of lower-level elements. Bergeron certainly thinks so, and even suggests that Wernicke must have been operating with an implicit understanding of the difference between a cognitive working and a cognitive use, the distinction that, as we saw in Chapter 3, Anderson made central to his original presentation of the massive redeployment hypothesis. If Bergeron's conjecture is correct, Wernicke's great methodological innovation—what set him apart from the phrenologists and even his predecessor Paul Broca, for example—consisted in his cautious reluctance to infer cognitive working (i.e., essential functional contribution across all task categories, considered in isolation of neural context) from cognitive use (i.e., high-level/gross cognitive function), an inference obviously susceptible to Poldrack's *reductio*.

In the same vein, the father of modern neuroscience and champion of the neuron doctrine, Santiago Ramón y Cajal, "was decidedly not a supporter of either the definition of psychological 'faculties' or their assignment to discrete, localized neural 'organs'" (Anderson 2014, p. xv):

> In [his] view, brain function is to be understood in terms of a hierarchy of reflexes, in the most sophisticated instances of which one responds not just to external but also to internal, and not just to current but also to stored stimuli. . . . In such a brain there can be no region for circumspection or poetic talent, for although a particular sensory experience or association may be stored in a particular place . . . the behavioral characteristics of the organism are realized only by the fluid activity of the whole system in its environment. (Anderson 2014, pp. xv–xvi)

The idea that specific circuits could be cued by various stimuli across both internal and external environments is a tolerably clear presage of the metamodal hypothesis of brain organization, which we encountered briefly in Chapter 2, and underwrites the possibility of neural reuse. (I revisit the metamodal hypothesis in more detail in the next chapter, as it bears greatly on the questions facing us there.)

4.2.2 Graph theory and network neuroscience

There is another usage of the term "module" that one often comes across in the literature. It is perhaps a testament to the immense versatility of modularity that it has descriptive utility well beyond the confines of cognitive science. Modules play an important role in fields as diverse as developmental and systems biology, ecology, mathematics, computer science, robotics, and industrial design. One interesting application of the term occurs in the study of networks, and neural networks in particular. Unfortunately, there is a danger of confusion here, because the network concept is significantly looser than the classical one in cognitive science. Thus it sometimes happens that different researchers, all of whom work in the cognitive sciences broadly speaking (including brain science), refer to "modularity" but mean different things by it.

A "network" is any organization with a weblike structure. The Internet, airline routes, food webs, and electrical grids spring immediately to mind, but these are only the most obvious examples among a great variety of phenomena displaying network design, including genetic regulation and protein interaction (Bullmore & Sporns 2012; Caldarelli & Catanzaro 2012, pp. 23–25). Networks manifest a number of important universal properties (Caldarelli & Catanzaro 2012, pp. 4–5). At the most elementary level, all networks comprise a collection of nodes (or "vertices") and the various connections (or "edges") between them (see Fig. 4.1). In a map of airline routes, for example, a single airport would be represented by a node and the route between any two of them by an edge. Because the focus of attention is the global structure of interactions between nodes, rather than the individual nodes themselves, the basic representational vehicle can be the same in every case; namely, a graph depicting nothing more than these nodes and their all-important interconnections (Caldarelli & Catanzaro 2012, pp. 4, 12; Anderson 2014, p. 12). In graph theory, a "module" is defined as a community of "densely interconnected nodes" where "the existence of several [such] communities is characteristic of [a] modular [network]" (Bullmore & Sporns 2012, p. 342; Caldarelli & Catanzaro 2012, pp. 89–90) (Fig. 4.1). In network neuroscience specifically, network models take the form of neural coactivation graphs, where modules are identified as communities of nodes that are functionally coactive (see later in this chapter). In the context of neural networks, then, "modularity refers to the existence of multiple communities of neurons or brain regions as defined by patterns of [functional] connectivity" (Bullmore & Sporns 2012, p. 342).

The point is explained very simply by Caldarelli & Catanzaro in connection with the importance of fMRI:

When humans perform an action, even one as simple as blinking, a storm of electrical signals from the neurons breaks out in several areas of the brain. These regions can be identified through techniques such as *functional*

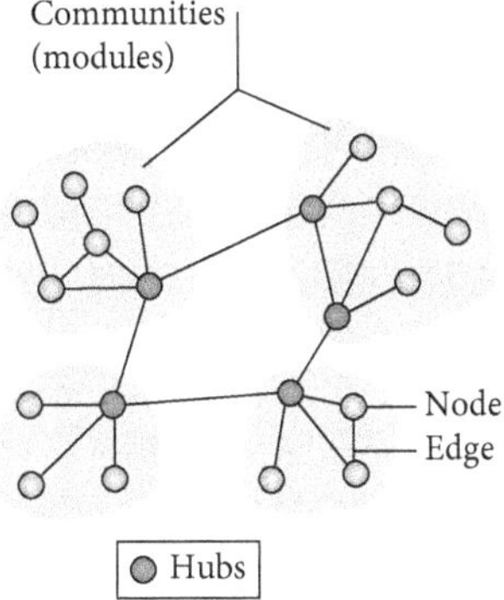

Figure 4.1 Nodes, edges, modules, and hubs in a network. Nodes are sometimes also called vertices.

(Reprinted by permission from Springer Nature, *Nature Reviews Neuroscience*, "The economy of brain network organization" by E. Bullmore and O. Sporns. Copyright 2018. Bullmore & Sporns 2018, p. 342.)

> *magnetic resonance.* Through this technique, scientists have discovered that different areas emit correlated signals. That is, they show a special synchronization that suggests that they may influence each other. (Caldarelli & Catanzaro 2012, p. 27)

Furthermore,

> These areas can be taken as nodes and an edge is drawn between two of them if there is a sufficient level of correlation. Also at this level, the brain appears as a set of connected elements [i.e., "modules"]. Each action of a person lights up a network of connected areas in the brain. (Caldarelli & Catanzaro 2012, p. 27)

That is, the neuroimaging data resulting from a functional connectivity analysis can be represented as a graph—a neural coactivation graph—in which nodes represent individual brain regions and edges denote the likelihood of coactivation between two nodes during a particular task (Anderson 2014, p. 12).

Why should this prove instructive for cognitive architecture? It turns out that the abstract topological features of these neural coactivation graphs frequently (if only roughly) track the functional taxonomies of cognitive psychology, cognitive neuropsychology, and the computationalist/functionalist tradition more generally (Anderson 2010, p. 303, 2014, p. 42). This sense of the word "module" therefore seems as if it might have a natural affinity with the modules to which philosophers of psychology have become accustomed. But closer inspection shows this to be a tentative link at best.

Firstly, being in effect sets of *reusable* (i.e., domain-general/task-selective) nodes, these graph-theoretical modules are not your typical dissociable ones (although see Pessoa 2016 for discussion); nor, for that matter, are they intended to track encapsulation, domain specificity, automaticity, or the half-dozen other features typically ascribed to modules within the computationalist tradition (Stanley & De Brigard 2016). Quite simply, the usage here is *sui generis*. Secondly, while there no doubt *is* a standard and more orthodox usage of the term "module" in neuroscience (one that moreover does offer some support to the classical conception from cognitive science, as I discuss later), its meaning is in fact much closer to what is represented by the nodes of a coactivation graph than by the *communities* of nodes in such a graph (see, e.g., Pascual-Leone & Hamilton 2001, p. 443; Pascual-Leone et al. 2005, p. 396; Caldarelli & Catanzaro 2012, p. 27; Fedorenko & Thompson-Schill 2014, pp. 120, 121; Zador 2015, p. 44). That is, the standard sense of "module" in neuroscience trails far more closely the idea of small, individual brain regions with discrete subfunctional profiles than it does the idea of high-level/gross-functional composites. The anomaly results from the fact that network techniques were developed independently of neuroscience and with a distinctive usage and vocabulary. When network methods were eventually adopted by neuroscientists, an idiosyncratic usage was introduced into a discipline that already had a fairly settled meaning for the term "module." In neuroscience, "module" typically refers to a cortical column (akin to a node in the coactivation graphs just discussed), and this, as we shall see further in §§ 4.3 and 5.1, is a twentieth-century refinement of the anatomical module within the structuralist tradition.

4.2.3 Separate modifiability as the touchstone of modularity

A common objection to accounts of cognitive architecture that downplay or question the modular hypothesis is that modularity has not been given due credit for the uniquely versatile concept that it is, and that the dissenters have simply fettered themselves with an impossibly narrow and needlessly structuralist conception of cognitive architecture that is unwarranted in all the circumstances (the circumstances being the Cognitive Revolution, the fact that no one seriously denies that the mind has a rich internal structure, the unquestionable boon of functional decomposition as an effective research strategy in the cognitive sciences, etc.). Jungé and Dennett (2010, p. 278) appear sympathetic to this point of view: "A software theory of massive modularity—programs evolved to serve particular adaptive functions within brains—without commitments about implementation (unlike anatomical modularity) could survive [*the evidence of neural reuse*] largely untouched." At issue here is whether a nondissociable system of some variety could be regarded as modular—whether, say, a language or norm acquisition device comprising very many smaller domain-general neural regions could in some sense be a module.[2] Against this suggestion is the claim that functional dissociability ought to fix a definite threshold beneath which a system cannot be regarded as modular. Here I shall contend for the latter view.

Recent developments in neuroscience have no doubt added to the luster of the "system" module, as I shall call it, and even encouraged the view that such modules represent what was always the most important contribution of modular theories to our understanding of the mind (see further in this chapter). But actually the system module has been around for a long time. Its fortunes can nowhere be more illuminatingly charted than in the annals of generative grammar. Generative grammarians are notorious for prevaricating on the issue of linguistic modularity—one can easily locate passages that would suggest the modularity in question is anatomical or at the very least functional (Chomsky 1975, pp. 40–41, 1980a, pp. 39, 44, 1988, p. 159, 2002, pp. 84–86; Pinker & Jackendoff 2005, p. 207; Fitch et al. 2005, p. 182; Collins 2008, p. 155), and others where what they seem to have in mind is little more than a "domain of inquiry"—"[t]he view that internal cognitive systems can fruitfully (for purposes of successful theory-construction) be studied independently of other such systems" (McGilvray 2014, p. 235; Chomsky 2005, p. 5). Notice that the module-as-domain-of-inquiry very effectively neutralizes the sting of neuroscientific evidence, since there is really no evidence that neuroscientists can adduce against the existence of such a module (a point to which I return later). Indeed, the system module is frequently endorsed by playing down the significance of implementation and

---

[2] In § 5.2, I consider whether it is possible for systems consisting of shared domain-general parts to be functionally dissociable. This is the same as asking whether higher-level/gross cognitive functions could persist as *functional* modules. For now, we can assume the answer is no.

emphasizing its "methodological value as a research heuristic" (Badcock et al. 2016, p. 11; see also Scholl 1997). But let us return to the other theme of this section, the notion of dissociability.

In a straightforward sense, a system is dissociable if it is functionally specialized—if it can (in principle) be modified without directly impeding the operation of a comparable system.[3] This is a matter of degree. So if a neural system n consisting of primitives $\{p_1, p_2, p_3 \ldots p_n\}$ contributes some specific and functionally discrete operation f such that any element of the set $\{p_1, p_2, p_3 \ldots p_n\}$ is dedicated to f, n will be *pro tanto* dissociable; the more elements in the set $\{p_1, p_2, p_3 \ldots p_n\}$ are dedicated to f, the more dissociable n will be.[4] On this understanding, a speech production center will be dissociable to the extent that its impairment has no direct effect on any system "considered with the same grain of analysis" (Carruthers 2008, p. 295) (e.g., numeracy, rhythm, speech comprehension, episodic memory, IQ, etc.), even though it might ramify to compromise a higher-level functional system that draws upon the speech production center for processing (e.g., singing, signing, etc.). In the context of neural reuse, we may presume that a working's impairment will ramify to all higher-level functional composites in which it plays an active role; and yet so long as no other *working* is directly put out by such an intervention, the working remains sufficiently discrete to be regarded as dissociable. (Whether brain regions as small as workings are *truly* dissociable in this sense is another question. I take it up in Chapter 5.)

Notice that when spelled out in this way—and all I have done is follow through with the logic of dissociability as it is commonly understood (see, e.g., Carruthers 2008, p. 258; Coltheart 2011, pp. 227–228)—the requirement could be thought to lose much of its explanatory power. For what it entails is that the smaller and more functionally promiscuous a neural system gets—remembering that neural reuse itself implies that the typical brain region will be both extremely small and highly versatile—the more difficult to quarantine the effects of regional impairment, since those effects will presumably ramify to all affected distributed systems. An evolutionary psychologist might allege that nothing theoretically significant can follow from the fact that a tiny brain region is dissociable if its impairment will disturb the operation of many higher-level cognitive systems. It is only when modules directly

---

[3] Its modification may of course *indirectly* impede a comparable "downstream" system; i.e., one at the receiving end of its efferent projections.

[4] What I am calling the "primitives" $\{p_1, p_2, p_3 \ldots p_n\}$ need not be neurons: they could be specific subneural processes or ions.

implement gross cognitive functions (e.g., sentence parsing, cheater detection, face recognition, and the like) that the effects of modification can be contained in a way that makes dissociability an important constraint on cognitive theory. For then evolution itself can have a clear role to play in shaping cognitive systems by selectively modifying brain regions in a way that does not reverberate detrimentally across distributed systems. This indeed was thought to be a major argument in favor of modularity—the neat solution it offered to the so-called evolutionary debugging problem (Cosmides & Tooby 1994). In contrast, any account of modularity in which modules come out as small and promiscuous is an account of modularity that no longer promises to solve the debugging problem. And (it may be alleged) any criterion of modularity that casts modules in such a diminutive role cannot be considered especially salient.

Now I am defending dissociability as a criterion of modularity. My position must therefore seem a little curious, for am I not by defending dissociability actually defending the wrong sorts of modules—given the sorts of modules that this criterion delivers if the redeployment hypothesis is correct? I can certainly see how an evolutionary psychologist would be puzzled by my position. But, as I shall explain later, I do not think the evolutionary psychologist's reasoning here is persuasive—frankly, the sorts of modules she is after are very unlikely to be found anywhere beyond the most primitive domains, and the search for them at all reflects a misunderstanding of the brain and its evolution: the debugging problem is not a deep one. Like it or not, therefore, it looks as if we are going to have to rest content with a diminutive role for modules—which may not be such a bad thing anyway. For while dissociability may not ultimately meet the desiderata for a theory of evolutionary psychology, it ought to safeguard a respectable threshold for modularity nonetheless. It furnishes a kind of cognitive "movable type" for the mind, and mechanisms that can support robust laws, generalizations, and predictions (e.g., "forward" inferences from cognitive tasks to brain areas) (Burnston 2016). If—

> for a given neural area A, there is some univocal description D, such that D explains the functional role of A's activity whenever A functions

—it should be possible to formulate a theory tokening A providing "functional descriptions that apply over a range of instances of functioning," and "functional explanations in particular contexts that are relevant to contexts not yet explored" (Burnston 2016, pp. 529, 531). This would be a "*very* powerful theor[y] in terms of generalizability and projectability" (Burnston 2016, p. 531).[5]

So what, then, of Jungé and Dennett's suggestion? The problem, as I see it, is that it confuses modularity with faculty psychology more generally, and so reduces it to a platitude. Being neither controversial, falsifiable, nor particularly interesting, the system view fails to live up to the theory's venerable reputation. On such an expansive definition, who would *not* emerge as a defender of modularity? Certainly few theorists in the cognitive neurosciences would deny the utility of functional decomposition as an effective research strategy (Prinz 2006; Piccinini & Craver 2011; Boone & Piccinini 2016).[6] And of course a higher-level cognitive system composed of shared neural elements might well exhibit natural kind properties, such as a systematic set of procedures for dealing with typical inputs (Chomsky 1980a; 2006; Pinker 1997). But it is difficult to see how such a definition could have any substantively worthwhile theoretical upshots, certainly of a kind that could possibly justify the enormous effort spent in advancing modularity as some sort of solution to a deep and longstanding set of issues. On this weak view, what would the modularity of cognition explain about cognition beyond the simple fact that the mind, too, may be investigated using the techniques of natural science (i.e., "divide and conquer" works here, too)? If the answer is "not much," this cannot be a good account of modularity—assuming that by "modularity" we mean a substantive doctrine. In the weak construal, modules turn out to be little more than fruitful perspectives on the mind, the mind considered from this or that particular point of view; say, the point of view of its linguistic capabilities, its pitch discrimination capabilities, its problem-solving

---

[5] Brain regions that are domain-general in the way envisaged by theories of neural reuse may of course ultimately prove *not* to sustain completely generalizable and projectable accounts of local function. The ability of a brain region to maintain a set of stable input-output relations, and hence to be truly dissociable, may be compromised by the effects of the neural network context. I pursue this topic in Chapter 5.

[6] Decomposability and modularity do come apart. Boone and Piccinini (2016, p. 1524) outline "a mechanistic version of homuncular functionalism, whereby higher-level cognitive capacities are iteratively explained by lower-level capacities until we reach a level in which the lower-level capacities are no longer cognitive in the relevant sense." While this might entail modularity for some lower-level elements (they do not say as much), it does not entail modularity for higher-level elements composed predominantly of shared parts (indeed, the word "modularity" or "module" appears nowhere in their paper): see McGeer's (2007) helpful discussion of the cognitive neuropsychologist's understanding of modularity. Prinz (2006) is actually explicit that, as long as the units of decomposition do not exhibit the properties associated with Fodorian modularity, we should proceed with decomposition but abandon the label of modularity. See my remarks, later in this chapter, for further clarification of this point.

capabilities, and so on (in principle, without limit). Such perspectives un-questionably give us useful entry points into what would otherwise be in-tractably complex, and allow us to figure out what it is that the mind actually does. But it is hardly surprising that a targeted coming-to-grips with a com-plex object should yield significant insights. The same strategy is familiar in one form or another in virtually all domains of rational inquiry, be they phys-ical, chemical, biological, psychological, or otherwise. That "science works here, too," I take not to be an interesting claim, if it comes to that, because it does not so much as provide a theory of cognition at all: if anything, it says more about science than it does about cognition. Furthermore, it is not en-tirely clear that the behaviorists would have spurned the sort of modules in view here. What they denied was the existence of *sui generis* principles, or the computational/architectural/modality independence of certain capaci-ties (e.g., language), which I regard as evidence of true modules. They would not as a rule have denied that a partition of their subject matter could lead to interesting results. Recall the title of Skinner's *Verbal Behavior*—I think it is fair to say that Skinner sought quite literally to explain *the language faculty*, albeit in terms of general associationist learning mechanisms, and is this not nearly comparable to the system sense of a module now under discussion? The behaviorists may have offered a shallow theory of human capacities, but even it did not appear to preclude modules in this sense (see, e.g., Chomsky 1979, pp. 49–51). Nor for that matter is there any logical reason why a connectionist or holist would have to rule them out, either. Contemporary Parallel Distributed Processing models of cognitive architecture in fact *do* have a sort of generic componential motivation behind them (O'Reilly 1998; Jilk et al. 2008).

It is worth being clear about exactly why system modularity fails the test of being "interesting." It is easy to be misled here by the genuinely "in-teresting" results that have been achieved as a consequence of adopting the system view; i.e., by what has been learned about distinct domains of psychology as a result of iterative functional analysis (task analysis, de-composition, "boxology," etc.). The system module's notable successes, as well as its historical association with the computational theory of mind and the view of the mind as richly and intricately structured, are apt to lead to an exaggerated estimate of its true significance. Any theory of the mind pitched at the level of faculties (or analyzable parts, components, units, etc.)—as modularity most assuredly is—must tell us what it does about the mind *through what it tells us about the faculties* (or whatever the relevant units of analysis happen to be). If it does not speak "through the faculties," as it were, it cannot so much as count as a faculty psychology, since the properties of the mind to which a faculty psychology brings our attention are, in the first instance, properties of the mind's faculties. This point is at once obvious and yet so readily overlooked that it needs to be emphasized. That the mind is richly structured, that the mind is a computer, that the mind obeys laws exhibiting a clear mathematical structure, and so forth—these statements, if they are true, are true of the mind *generally*, meaning that it ought to be unsurprising if the *divisions* of the mind are correspondingly rich, intricate, computational, systematic, and so on. None of these properties attach to faculties *per se*. Moreover, learning that the *language* faculty has such-and-such features, or that *vision* operates in this or that fashion, need not tell us much about faculties *qua* faculties either, as against telling us about this or that particular faculty. Thus neither *general* claims about the mind associated with the Cognitive Revolution, nor *specific* claims about *specific* faculties, hard-won though these insights may have been, automatically get reckoned as among the distinctive insights marking out a truly *general theory* of faculties, which is after all what a faculty psychology aims to be. Contrast such claims with those of a well-developed faculty psychology (e.g., Fodor 1983). The roster of properties associated with Fodorian modularity (domain specificity; encapsulation; shallow, fast, and mandatory processing; hardwiredness; etc.) do not amount to a list of properties pertaining to the mind generally, nor to specific faculties considered independently, but to *all* faculties *qua* faculties. This is what made his theory interesting. So, as easy as it is to roll the system module in the glitter of the Cognitive Revolution, a frank assessment of this module demands that we isolate clearly what it is the theory that posits such modules says about the mind *at the level of faculties*—and when we do this, I maintain, we will be hard put to find anything that would not heartily be conceded by anyone who believes in the power of science (be they classical modularists, connectionists, holists, and, as I suggested, probably even behaviorists, *mutatis mutandis*).

Furthermore, lest it be thought that the very idea of functional decomposition can underwrite the system view—for one must admit that decomposition proceeds in a curious fashion where computers are concerned; namely, via the execution of subroutines by simpler algorithms or subagencies ("homunculi"), surely a nontrivial design feature of such systems—it need only be pointed out that *homuncularity* is not the same as *modularity*. Careful psychologists have always understood the difference, and that modularity is really a special type of homuncularity (Mahon & Cantlon 2011, pp. 149–151), just as homuncularity is a special type of decomposition (van Gelder 1995, p. 351). It is interesting to observe in this connection that David Marr, one of the chief architects of the computational theory of mind, did not see computationalism (and therefore, we may surmise, homuncular functionalism) as providing a free pass to his "principle of modular design." Modularity seems for Marr to be an added feature that *some* computational systems, for largely heuristic reasons, might be thought to possess:

> Any large computation should be split up and implemented as a collection of small sub-parts that are as nearly independent of one another as the overall task allows. If a process is not designed in this way, a small change in one place will have consequences in many other places. This means that the process as a whole becomes extremely difficult to debug or to improve, whether by a human designer or in the course of natural evolution, because a small change to improve one part has to be accompanied by many simultaneous compensating changes elsewhere. (Marr 1976, p. 485)

So, although homuncularity is not so generic as "mere decomposition," it is nowhere near as important a principle as modularity, either. Accordingly (and for additional reasons I canvass later), we should withhold the more serious designation from generic system subcomponents and procedures that are non-dissociable.

So far, I have said nothing about two important features of classically modular systems: domain specificity and informational encapsulation. Can they get the system module over the line? Actually, the question itself is incoherent. Consider that once a module is allowed to consist of shared parts, it can no longer be domain-specific, except perhaps in an abstract sense (see § 7.2.1). This is because the "module" will be sensitive to potentially many domains, since its parts are presumably domain-general (see § 4.3). Put another way, domain specificity[7] requires a functionally integrated unit that can respond to specified inputs. While the component modules of a composite consisting of shared parts would be functionally integrated, it is not

---

[7] Of whatever variety—strict or formal (see §§ 2.4.3 and 5.1).

obvious that the composite itself would be, although it might be said to have a sort of ad hoc integrity when in use. Notice also that a composite is unlikely to be informationally encapsulated "precisely because in sharing parts [it] will have access to the information stored and manipulated by [other high-level systems]" (Anderson 2010, p. 300). Anatomically distributed and overlapping brain networks simply must share information on some level (Pessoa 2016, p. 23). Lacking both of these properties, then, one or the other of which has been considered definitive (Coltheart 1999; Fodor 1983, p. 71), its postulation does not quite serve the purposes many would assume. One might have supposed that the system module could be more strongly motivated if at least it had the property of either domain specificity or encapsulation (in a concrete and unambiguous sense). And yet just *because* it is a composite, it can be neither truly domain-specific nor (in all likelihood) informationally encapsulated.

In something of a *reductio*, then, the system view of modularity leads only to the claim that the mind can do different things at different times. Certainly a more ambitious and theoretically interesting claim than this is available; namely, that the mind can do different things at the *same* time; but as far as we know this requires functional specialization; i.e., separate moving parts (*real* modules), since the prospect of neural time-sharing appears low (see § 7.5 on the time-sharing problem). The pervasiveness of cognitive interference effects and processing bottlenecks in stimulus-rich environments that impose overwhelming attentional demands is enough to make this clear (Anderson 2010, p. 250). In short, either these debates are trifling, or the claims at stake are more adventurous than the system view permits. Here I shall presume that the more adventurous reading is correct, and that, in any event, functional dissociability really ought to be considered the *sine qua non* of modularity.

Bear in mind also that, in the context of cognitive neuropsychology, modules have been defined largely by reference to what the dissociation evidence has revealed; i.e., "on the basis of the specific behavioral effects of brain lesions" (Bergeron 2007, p. 177). Bergeron calls this inferential strategy the "functional modularity inference." Basically, "the presence of highly selective cognitive impairments (dissociations) like prosopagnosia and various linguistic processing deficits suggest [*sic*] the functional independence of at least some cognitive processes," and this in turn licenses the postulation of functionally independent modules subserving those processes (Bergeron 2007, pp. 176, 177; Gazzaniga 1989, p. 147). The fact that brain lesions are often also relatively localized suggests that such modules reside in a "specific and relatively small portion of the brain" (the "anatomical modularity inference") (Bergeron 2007, p. 176; Gazzaniga 1989, pp. 947, 950). Make no mistake, the legitimacy of these inferences is hotly contested, since noisy dissociations are compatible with a system's being dissociable, and clean dissociations compatible with a system's being substantially nondissociable. In the first instance, "there are a variety of reasons, well explored in the neuropsychology literature, for which lesions to brain systems can produce noisy rather than clean patterns of breakdown even when the systems required to complete the task are modular" (Barrett & Kurzban 2006, p. 642). A good example would be a focal lesion at the border of two adjacent modules—the breakdown would not be clean, yet the two systems would be modular. In the second instance, even perfect (or "double") dissociations cannot conclusively establish that the affected systems are modular, for a lesion might only compromise a small isolable component of an otherwise highly interpenetrative circuit. Damage to this component might result in the system depending on that component being independently impaired, but it does not follow from this that the system would be functionally dedicated (although admittedly it would be dissociable at the margins). In light of this, it may come as something of a surprise to be told that these arguments

> have failed to deter theorists from employing either of the inferential strategies. Indeed, the functional modularity inference continues to be one of the most common approaches among cognitive neuropsychologists for inquiring about the structure of cognition. Similarly, the recent cognitive neuroscience literature abounds more than ever with cases involving the use of the anatomical modularity inference. (Bergeron 2007, p. 177)

But what the persistence of these inferences bears witness to is the fundamental role that dissociation evidence plays in the search for modules, and that functional specificity itself continues to be the lodestar for deciding upon whether, and if so to what extent, the mind is modular within the major disciplinary fields concerned with this question. As we have seen, the same assumption underwrites evolutionary psychology and massive modularity, the central claim of which is that the mind is predominantly composed of parts selectively shaped by evolutionary pressures (Carruthers 2006). As two prominent evolutionary psychologists state their position (Barrett &

Kurzban 2006, p. 630): "... we intend an explicitly evolutionary reading of the concepts of function and specialization: modules evolved through a process of descent with modification, due to the effects they had on an organism's fitness." This view predicates the existence of systems that, though perhaps spatially extended and neurally interspersed, are dissociable in principle:

> Psychologists generally agree—as do we—that because cognitive architecture is instantiated in brain architecture, the two will be isomorphic at some level. . . . However, at a larger, macroscopic level, there is no reason to assume that there must be spatial units or chunks of brain tissue that neatly correspond to information-processing units. An analogy might be to the wiring in a stereo, a computer, or other electronic system: Individual wires have specific functions, but at the level of the entire machine, wires with different functions might cross and overlap. For this reason, removing, say, a three-inch square chunk from the machine would not necessarily remove just one of the machine's functions and leave the rest intact. In brain terms, it could be, and probably is, that macroscopic regions of brain tissue include neurons from multiple information-processing systems with multiple functions. (Barrett & Kurzban 2006, p. 641)

And of course other contemporary models of cognitive architecture, such as the successful ACT-R model, also posit the existence of independently modifiable subsystems of the brain.

When it comes to clarifying just what makes modularity interesting, one final set of considerations may be suggestive. While terminological nuances can hardly be decisive in an area like this, I think it is no coincidence that massive modularity bottoms out in claims about the separate modifiability of functional components. This is because the very word "module" evokes images of movable parts that can be assembled and reassembled in a variety of distinct combinations and that may be affected independently of one another. If all modularity amounts to is the claim that the mind can do different things at different times (rather than the stronger claim that it can do different things at the *same* time), and this suffices to call it "modular," it ought to be permissible to say that a knife that cuts both meat and bread is modular. And yet no one thinks of knives as modular (unless they are Swiss Army knives, which actually come with different blades). It is, I think, instructive that other anatomically nondissociable systems with shared parts, such as nervous systems, reproductive systems, endocrine systems, and the like—all of which may be singled out for their natural kind properties—*are* termed "systems." One never hears of digestive modules or reproductive modules. The "modules" of developmental biology and neuroscience that do have shared and reusable elements are an anomaly of network science. Most biologists, including developmental biologists, continue to think of modules as "anatomically distinct parts that can evolve independently" (Wolpert 2011, p. 115). Limbs and vertebrae would be modular on this view (being organs), but not the larger anatomical systems they compose.

It is well worth stressing here that my argument should not be read as an instance of mere carping or terminological pedantry. There are certainly occasions when scruples over the use of words reveal carping tendencies, and nothing much beyond that, but this is not one of them. Philosophers and cognitive scientists who allege a "module" for this capacity and a "module" for that capacity must be taken to be saying something substantial; i.e., something more than merely the fact that we *have* the capacities in question. To dignify these capacities with the honorific title "module" is, I would suggest, an attempt to invest the capacities with special-purpose, special-structure status. If philosophers and cognitive scientists persist in referring to modules for X and Y in the face of contrary evidence (i.e., evidence suggesting that the X and Y "modules" are not special-purpose, special-structure devices), they betray a willingness to exploit the connotations of a powerful term for rhetorical purposes. For, if by alleging that there is a module for X or Y the speaker intends only to say that we can give systematic accounts of X and Y—where X and Y represent particular foci of the scientific gaze upon the mind—the speaker is only avowing a belief in the efficacy of the scientific method in the realm of cognition, which I take it no naturalist would deny. In such circumstances, it would be better to drop the term "module" altogether, and settle for a less loaded (and therefore more honest) term like "capacity," "faculty," or "system."

So, while it is true that I am insisting on correct usage, this insistence is not without justification, and not without consequences should laxity prevail. In some ways the issues here are analogous to those that have arisen in the philosophy of biology over the proper use of the word "innate" (see Chapter 6). Neither those who urge elimination—because the word engenders confusion and fallacies of ambiguity amid a plethora of conflicting folk-biological intuitions—nor those arguing that a technical definition can be given should be seen as engaging in a merely feeble semantic dispute.

4.3 The Brain Module

As I have already mentioned several times in passing, neuroscience gets by for the most part with a very specific notion of modularity at hand. This is not the sense in which modules are familiar in network science, nor the sense in which they are familiar in most of psychology and cognitive science. The neuroscientific module is sometimes called a "brain module" or "cortical module" (Mountcastle 1978, 1997; Pascual-Leone & Hamilton 2001; Gold & Roskies 2008; Rowland & Moser 2014; Zador 2015), at other times a "cortical column" or "columnar module" (Mountcastle 1978, 1997; Buxhoeveden & Casanova 2002; Amaral & Strick 2013; Zador 2015), still at other times an "elementary processing unit" (Kandel & Hudspeth 2013), or simply an "operator" (Pascual-Leone & Hamilton 2001; Pascual-Leone et al. 2005). As I foreshadowed earlier, it corresponds (very roughly) with the node of a neural coactivation graph.[8] Slight variations in the meanings of these terms will not be important in the present context. It is true that the cortical "column" forms part of a distinctive hypothesis in neuroscience that arguably contemplates a narrower class of phenomena than is conveyed by the nodes of a network graph. But nothing need turn on this here. Indeed, from one point of view, the metamodal (reusable) node is a fully generalized account of the more specific columnar module (Jacobs 1999, pp. 33–34; Pascual-Leone & Hamilton 2001, pp. 427–428, 441, 443).

Various formulations of the criteria for modularity have been proposed in neuroscience (Buxhoeveden & Casanova 2002, p. 940). The general notion is of a coherent functional unit with a more or less dedicated input–output specification, somewhat on a par with the modern microprocessor chip (Leise 1990, p. 1). Gazzaniga (1989, p. 947) assumes "a high degree of functional specificity in the information transmitted over neural systems," and that modular organization consists of "identifiable component processes that participate in the generation of a cognitive state. The effects of *isolating* entire modular systems or of *disconnecting* the component parts can be observed" (my emphasis). Leise (1990) defines "module" as a group of cells with similar

---

[8] Of course, what corresponds to a node in network neuroscience is somewhat arbitrary. For certain purposes, neuroscientists may use a neuroanatomically delimited region as a node, whereas for other purposes they may use another one. I certainly would not wish to say that a module is something that depends on the interest of the neuroscientist. (I thank an anonymous reviewer for bringing this point to my attention.) Additionally, the notion of a "module" in network neuroscience is, as we saw in Chapter 4, different from the notion of a "node." A module in network theory refers to a *community* of nodes.

response properties (see also Amaral & Strick 2013, p. 348; Zador 2015, p. 44). Krubitzer (1995, p. 412) defines them as "structural and physiological discontinuities within the limits of a classically defined cortical field . . . reflected in architectonic appearance . . . neural-response properties, stimulus preference and connections." The idea here is clearly predicated upon both functional and anatomical specificity.

The brain module's explanatory rationale is simple. As Gazzaniga (1989, p. 947) concludes from a review of the comparative evidence, "research on animals has led to the belief that there are anatomic modules involved in information processing of all kinds and that they work in parallel and are distributed throughout the brain." In the same vein, Kandel and Hudspeth (2013, p. 17) state that neuroscientists "now think that all [higher level] cognitive abilities result from the interaction of many processing mechanisms distributed in several regions of the brain. Specific brain regions are *not responsible for specific mental faculties*" (my emphasis). Higher level/gross functions such as language, perception, affect, thought, movement, and memory "are all made possible by the *interlinkage* of serial and parallel processing in *discrete* brain regions, each with *specific* functions" (Kandel & Hudspeth 2013, p. 17, my emphasis; Bressler 1995; Gazzaniga 1989, p. 947). High-level mental functions fractionate into low-level subfunctions, then, and it is these narrowly defined low-level operating systems that are understood to satisfy the criteria for modularity in neuroscience. The key principle here is that of *distributed parallel processing*, in which "functional parts . . . interconnect uniquely to form processing networks" (Krubitzer 1995, p. 408; Bressler 1995; Mountcastle 1997, p. 717). Kandel and Hudspeth give a vivid illustration:

> Simple introspection suggests that we store each piece of our knowledge as a single representation that can be recalled by memory-jogging stimuli or even by the imagination alone. Everything you know about your grandmother, for example, seems to be stored in one complete representation that is equally accessible whether you see her in person, hear her voice, or simply think about her. Our experience, however, is not a faithful guide to how knowledge is stored in memory. Knowledge about grandmother is not stored as a single representation but rather is subdivided into distinct categories and stored separately. One region of the brain stores information about the invariant physical features that trigger your visual recognition of her. Information about changeable aspects of her face—her expression and

lip movements that relate to social communication—is stored in another region. The ability to recognize her voice is mediated in yet another region. (2013, pp. 17–18)

This picture fits flush with the sort of distributed parallel activation evidence that underpins neural reuse (Pasqualotto 2016; Pessoa 2016). Indeed, to the extent that they are not strictly domain-specific, the stable low-level operations that occur as nodes in these distributed systems seem to be the empirical equivalent of the low-level cognitive workings posited in the earliest formulations of the massive redeployment hypothesis.

A little history will clarify the significance of this discovery. The elaboration of the distributed processing model is the high point of an intense research effort within the structuralist tradition. In my earlier discussion, I noted that Carl Wernicke stood out among the ranks of modern neurologists with his distinctive vision of the structure–function relationship. I suggested that he may even have been operating with an implicit understanding of the difference between a cognitive working and a cognitive use (Bergeron 2007). In a famous paper, Wernicke (1908) described a novel kind of aphasia, one in which the patient can produce words but not comprehend them—the precise inverse of the pathology described by Broca earlier that century. The brain lesion responsible for this aphasia was to a distinct cortical region of the left cerebral hemisphere (later called "Wernicke's area"). Wernicke presented his account of this pathology in terms of an explicit neural model of language processing that attempted to steer a middle course between the two competing frameworks of his day, that of the phrenologists and cellular connectionists on one hand, who contended that specific functions were realized in localized neural tissue (and were therefore guided by the anatomical modularity assumption), and that of the holists on the other, who supposed that every mental function involved the brain as an aggregate (Kandel & Hudspeth 2013). Wernicke's model had only basic sensory-motor and perceptual functions localized to discrete regions of cortex. Higher functions depended on the cooperation of several neural elements, implying that single behaviors could not be pinned down to specific sites. Wernicke thus became the first neurologist to advance the thoroughly modern notion of distributed processing (Kandel & Hudspeth 2013; Mountcastle 1997). He assigned a specific language motor program governing the mouth movements for speech to the region implicated in Broca's aphasia, and a sensory program governing word perception to the area implicated in the new aphasia he described.

According to this model, the initial steps in neural processing of spoken or written words occur in separate sensory areas of the cortex specialized for auditory or visual information. This information is then conveyed to a cortical association area, the angular gyrus, specialized for processing both auditory and visual information. Here, according to Wernicke, spoken or written words are transformed into a neural sensory code shared by both speech and writing. This representation is conveyed to Wernicke's area, where it is recognized as language and associated with meaning. It is also relayed to Broca's area, which contains the rules, or grammar, for transforming the sensory representation into a motor representation that can be realized as spoken or written language. When this transformation from sensory to motor representation cannot take place, the patient loses the ability to speak and write. (Kandel & Hudspeth 2013, p. 12)

The success of Wernicke's clinical model in predicting a third type of aphasia—one in which "the receptive and expressive zones for speech are intact, but the neuronal fibers that connect them are destroyed"—as well as its general influence among late–nineteenth-century neurologists, helped inaugurate a new approach to cortical localization spearheaded by the German anatomist Korbinian Brodmann. Brodmann's revolutionary method of distinguishing cortical regions on the basis of cellular shape and vertical orientation brings us one step closer to the cortical columns that are now taken to be the "fundamental computational modules of the neocortex" (Amaral & Strick 2013, p. 348).

Brodmann's contribution was to extend the histological and cytoarchitectonic methods of his day by working comparatively; i.e., across species. He showed that neurons in the cerebral cortex have both a layer-wise (laminar) and vertical (columnar) orientation, and used this structure to guide his subdivision of the brain into more functionally discrete regions. Specifically, Brodmann noted differences in the packing densities and shapes of neurons as he bored down into the cortex, as well as differences in laminar thickness and synaptic connections as he traveled horizontally along its surface. This proved to be a decisive step, for we now know that functional differences in cortex depend on the relative thickness of layers as one moves from region to region. Each of its six layers is characterized by different inputs and outputs, with neurons projecting to different parts of the brain. "Projections to other parts of the neocortex, the so-called cortico-cortical or associational connections, arise primarily from neurons in layers II and III. Projections to subcortical regions arise mainly from layers V and VI" (Amaral & Strick 2013, p. 346). "Input" areas such as the primary visual cortex receive sensory information from the thalamus, and therefore have an enlarged layer IV, since this is where axons from the thalamus typically terminate: "The input layer contains a specialized type of excitatory neuron called the stellate cell, which has a dense bushy dendrite that is relatively localized, and seems particularly good at collecting the local axonal input to this layer" (O'Reilly et al. 2012, p. 33). "Hidden" areas, processing neither inputs nor outputs but essential to the formation of abstract category representations, are thickest at layers II and III, since the predominance of pyramidal cells in these layers makes them "well positioned for performing this critical categorization function" (O'Reilly et al. 2012, p. 34). Finally, "output" areas have their thickest layers at layers V and VI, given that the efferent connections that typify output zones must "synapse directly onto [subcortical] muscle control areas," and it is the neurons in these layers that best meet this requirement (O'Reilly et al. 2012, p. 34). Brodmann marked the boundaries where these surface differences occurred and was thus able to distinguish the 47 distinct brain regions that have since become eponymous. Each of Brodmann's brain areas consequently relates to a specific cognitive or sensory-motor function: areas 44 and 45, for instance, correspond to Broca's area, and area 22 corresponds to Wernicke's area.

This is where modules reenter the story. The sort of cytoarchitectonic methods that Brodmann employed, while delivering a very useful functional subdivision by the standards of his day, were not quite able to do justice to the subtlety of functional variation in the cortex. For the five regions Brodmann designated as being concerned with visual function (areas 17–21), modern electrophysiological and connectional analyses have interposed 35. These take the form of cortical columns that run from the outermost surface of the cortical sheet (the so-called *pial* surface) to the white matter deep beneath layer VI. A "column" is in effect a very thin cross-sectional slice of the cortical field, no more than a fraction of a millimeter across, such that "[n]eurons within a column tend to have very similar response properties, presumably because they form a local processing network" (Amaral & Strick 2013, p. 348). It is this distinctive columnar structure that passes for the basic cognitive module of neuroscience today (Mountcastle 1997; Zador 2015), and its importance resides, partly at least, in the computational efficiency it confers on neural circuits:

> Columnar organization . . . minimizes the distance required for neurons
> with similar functional properties to communicate with one another and
> allows them to share inputs from discrete pathways that convey infor-
> mation about particular sensory attributes. This efficient connectivity
> economizes on the use of brain volume and maximizes processing speed.
> The clustering of neurons into functional groups, as in the columns of the
> cortex, allows the brain to minimize the number of neurons required for
> analyzing different attributes. If all neurons were tuned for every attribute,
> the resultant combinatorial explosion would require a prohibitive number
> of neurons. (Gilbert 2013, p. 570)

At least part of the motivation for the brain module, then, is to address
concerns pertaining to the scaling problem we encountered in § 3.2 (i.e.,
as the number of neurons increases, the number of neurons that must be
connected grows quadratically larger). It is genuinely modular in the sense of
possessing both functional specificity—i.e., a discrete computational operation definable over a preferred (but nonexclusive) set of inputs—and spatial
localization (Pascual-Leone & Hamilton 2001, pp. 441, 443; Gazzaniga 1989,
p. 947; O'Reilly et al. 2012, pp. 36–40; Pasqualotto 2016; Pessoa 2016).

All this is predominantly (and paradigmatically) true of the sensory-motor
cortical maps discussed in Chapter 2. Many of these have "functionally specific, connected neurons to extract behaviorally relevant features [e.g., lines
and edges from spatial receptive fields] from incoming sensory information" and "a degree of functional autonomy" (Rowland & Moser 2014, p. 22).
Whether this organization is exemplified also by non-sensory/non-motor
high-end association cortices has not up until now been clear, but Rowland
and Moser (2014) review evidence suggesting that there are definite similarities between sensorimotor columns and the organization found in me-
dial entorhinal cortex (MEC) implicated in episodic and spatial memory
tasks. If the grid map of MEC really were to be organized in this modular
fashion, it would certainly put paid to the idea of a rigid Cartesian distinction between "central" and "peripheral" cognition as far as modularity is concerned (see § 7.2.2). Of course, the precise degree to which MEC resembles
columnar organization is the crucial question. The similarities for their part
are clear: MEC has "vertically linked cells, tight bundling of dendrites from
the deeper layers, and predominantly local connections raising the possibility that it contains functionally autonomous columns" (Rowland & Moser
2014, p. 22). Moreover, "MEC has well-defined spatial responses that allow

the cells to be analyzed for topography and modularity in their response properties" (Rowland & Moser 2014, p. 22). There *is* one noteworthy difference, however. The majority of entorhinal modules appear to be anatomically intermingled such that, while they remain functionally independent and discrete (dissociable in principle), they are anatomically overlapping and spatially interspersed, rather than strictly localized. Entorhinal modules therefore appear to be merely functional, not anatomical. Their functional specificity is further corroborated by the fact that, although columns are themselves composed of far smaller units called "minicolumns" (consisting of between 80 and 100 neurons), "[n]o research has yet determined the capacity of minicolumns for independent activity outside the macrocolumn that they belong to" (Buxhoeveden & Casanova 2002, p. 937). The upshot of all this is that the brain could be organized into column-based modules of roughly common form throughout, including regions that are important to central cognition.

What needs most emphasizing about the brain module are the very qualities that set it apart from the classical notion that still features unmistakably in discussions of modularity within cognitive science, cognitive neuropsychology, neuropsychology, and the philosophy of mind. Here I am referring to its extremely restricted scope—an exiguously small subfunctional computation—and its dynamic metamodal response properties: the brain module is in essence a domain-general reusable operator appearing within various interacting, nested, and distributed neural assemblies (Mountcastle 1997; Jacobs 1999; Pascual-Leone & Hamilton 2001, Pascual-Leone et al. 2005; Pasqualotto 2016; Pessoa 2016). We saw these dynamic response properties in connection with an earlier discussion revolving around crossmodal plasticity, supramodal organization, and domain specificity (§§ 2.4.2–2.4.3). I shall revisit and elaborate on this material in the next section, when I explain more fully the character and import of Pascual-Leone and Hamilton's (2001) original metamodal hypothesis of brain organization. It will be relevant both to the issue of the functional specificity of modules (§ 5.1) and to their early development (Chapter 6).

Thus far I have provided an outline of the varieties of modularity, defended what I take to be indispensable in any modular theory of the mind, and foregrounded the neuroscientific notion of modularity. The next chapter pursues head-on the implications of neural reuse for the modularity of mind.

4.4 Summary

In recent decades, neuroscience has challenged the orthodox account of the modular mind. As I have shown, one way of meeting this challenge has been to go for increasingly "soft" versions of modularity, and one version in particular, which I dub the "system" view, is so soft that it promises to meet practically any challenge neuroscience can throw at it. But an account of the mind that tells us that the mind can do different things, even interesting things, is not itself necessarily an interesting account. In this chapter, I have reconsidered afresh what we ought to regard as the *sine qua non* of modularity, and offered a few arguments against the view that an insipid "system" module could be the legitimate successor of the traditional notion. In part my arguments can be read as a plea for the precise use of language, but there is more than pettifogging behind this plea.

5

Modules Reconsidered

Whither Modularity?

5.1 Does Modularity Survive the Evidence of Neural Reuse?

One of the primary contentions of this chapter is that the cortical column we have just examined is probably the only robust example of modularity that *could* survive evidence of reuse, and this just because reuse seems almost destined to predict something very much like it: small, stable, reusable nodes appearing within various distributed networks spanning various cognitive domains. The question before us now is whether despite appearances, neural redeployment really *is* compatible with the degree of functional specificity that modularity demands.

One thing appears reasonably certain. If the cortical column (or Andersonian "working") were to survive reuse as the dedicated and functionally specific cognitive unit that it would need to be, not only would reuse then be compatible with the modularity of mind, it seems fair to say the Fodorian module itself would be likely to survive in some form—at least to the extent that cortical columns retain both stimulus specificity and informational autonomy, properties that they are likely to retain if brain regions are as task-selective and functionally constrained as the evidence in § 2.4.3 suggests they are. To be sure, the neo-Fodorian module would be a shadow of its former self, barely recognizable in size and certainly no longer suited to its original role as a marker of gross cognitive function.[1] But the resulting picture of the mind would still be modular.

---

[1] For a similar criticism of Fodor's module, see Arbib (1989). Note that, by describing Fodor's modules as marking "gross" functions, I mean only that they can be specified at the level of proprietary domains (e.g., at the level of vision, olfaction, and aspects of language comprehension) rather than simply at the level of edge-detection or depth discrimination. They are not high-level in the sense that they pertain to complex thought, judgment, or memory. See § 7.2.2 for comment on Fodor's central/peripheral distinction.

But *does* the cortical column—or its Andersonian concomitant—emerge unscathed in this way? To get a sharper sense of the options available to us on this question, I shall set the overall account of reuse in the context of Pascual-Leone and Hamilton's (2001) original metamodal hypothesis, which is an important forerunner of contemporary theories of reuse, including Anderson's. This account trades in brain modules, which it terms "operators," and so allows me to convey very crisply the obvious sense in which modularity is compatible with reuse. I shall then walk through the principal objections to this view. Given what I take modules to be, my criterion of demarcation must be the degree to which dissociability no longer remains tenable even in principle. If functional specificity is no more than a will-o'-the-wisp, modularity itself can be little more than that. Therefore, I shall propose a simple device by which we can usefully conceptualize the problem facing the modularist. At its core, modularity turns on evidence of specialization. What we require, then, is a scale of specificity for brain regions that makes their indicia of specificity explicit. To the best of my knowledge, such indicia have not been presented in quite the same way before.[2] I conclude this section with an assessment of the long-run prospects of modularity.

The metamodal hypothesis is intended to account for the observation that "our perceptual experience of the world is richly multimodal"—that "[w]e are able to extract information derived from one sensory modality and use it in another," and "know a shape by touch and identify it correctly by sight" (Pascual-Leone & Hamilton 2001, p. 427). The hypothesis accommodates the possibility of crossmodal recruitment, and more specifically, the supramodal dynamics we encountered in § 2.4.3. Of relevance here is the fact that it is an adaptation of Robert Jacobs's (1999) "mixtures of experts" (ME) model. The ME model builds on two important ideas. First is the idea of functional specificity and spatial localization (i.e., the anatomical modularity assumption). Different brain regions possess different structural properties, and these differences make for differences in functional capability to the extent that some regions will be better suited to performing particular functions than others. Second is the idea of competition between modules. Brain regions become specialized for processing particular inputs through open

---

[2] I hasten to add, however, that Anderson's (2014) "dispositional vector" account of brain regions is an alternative strategy for coming to grips with the same set of issues. Others are clearly alive to the problem. Proponents of the Leabra architecture, for instance, resist modularist terminology precisely because it "forces a binary distinction on what is fundamentally a continuum" (Petrov et al. 2010, p. 287). See also Frost et al. (2015).

competition, but the competition is rigged, as it were, by the functional proficiencies that characterize the different regions: "each region tends to win the competition for those functions for which its structure makes it particularly well suited" (Jacobs 1999, p. 32). Two predictions follow. One is that the differences between neural regions appear quite early in development, and might even be innate (an issue to which I return in Chapter 6). The other is that "neural modules should enforce the outcome of a competition through a set of adaptable inhibitory interactions that allow modules to suppress the outputs of other modules" (Jacobs 1999, p. 34). Accordingly, Pascual-Leone and Hamilton propose that, instead of "unimodal sensory systems that are eventually integrated in multimodal association cortical regions," the *whole* cortex

> might actually represent a metamodal structure organized as operators that execute a given function or computation regardless of sensory input modality. Such operators might have a predilection for a given sensory input based on its relative suitability for the assigned computation. Such predilection might lead to operator-specific selective reinforcement of certain sensory inputs, eventually generating the impression of a brain structured in parallel segregated systems processing different sensory signals. In this view, the "visual cortex" is only "visual" because we have sight, and because the assigned computation of the striate cortex is best accomplished using retinal, visual information. Similarly, the "auditory cortex" is only auditory in hearing individuals and only because the computation performed by the temporal, perisylvian cortex is best implemented on cochlear, auditory signals. However, in the face of visual deprivation, the "striate cortex operator" will unmask its tactile and auditory inputs to implement its assigned computation using the available sensory information. (2001, pp. 427–428)

The crucial message for us here is that in this picture, despite neural operators being functionally and computationally constrained, their range of application is not. Neural operators are intrinsically versatile from the point of view of which inputs they can process, limited only by the amenability of the inputs to undergo a definite sort of manipulation. Barrett and Kurzban (2006, pp. 634–635) call something like this *formal* domain specificity—a construal of domain specificity wherein "domain" is not understood semantically, as referring to the set of objects or stimuli comprising a traditional task category, but rather *syntactically*, as the formal processing competence of a system. Formal domain specificity (essentially domain generality) comports with a view of the brain in which its several regions have manifold latent afferent input channels—preexisting connections supplying the critical cortical infrastructure that makes reuse possible. And while the picture presented in the preceding quotations would suggest a certain stability or equilibrium is achieved after a suppression mechanism ensures that the best module wins (so that individual modules get tuned to particular inputs and not others), as the examples presented in Chapter 2 dramatically attest, we do not have to wait for "visual deprivation" for this hidden complexity to be "unmasked," since it is a normal feature of healthy adult brains to exploit these channels all the time (e.g., when "seeing" the face of a loved one at the sound of their voice, or tools at the sound of a hammer, etc.). Hence, supramodal organization simply entails neural reuse. Moreover, the model demonstrates how readily modularity can be combined with redeployment, inasmuch as the latter naturally presupposes the former.

But now we must finally confront the objections to this "minimodule" view that reuse seems to entail. We can distinguish two broad lines of attack: one weak, the other far more serious and potentially fatal. It is well to address the weaker one first. Here the charge is that minimodules are "compatible with an anemic version of localization that claims simply that individual brain areas do something, and the same thing, however low-level, simple, or cognitively uninteresting, whenever they are activated" (Anderson 2007c, p. 164). Such entities can hardly be controversial, since very few people nowadays regard the brain as a "disorganized mash" (Prinz 2006). Notice that this is the same objection I raised earlier against the system view of modularity: "when the notion of modularity is denatured, it turns into a platitude" (Prinz 2006). And for all their differences, neither systems nor minimodules pretend to solve the evolutionary debugging problem. So we seem to have another case of truism dressed up as theory.

In the case of minimodules, however, I think the objection can be overplayed. It is true that minimodules are incapable of offering a simple way through the debugging problem, and this might be thought to commend the sort of modules defended by evolutionary psychologists instead. But what would be the use of a theory that resolved puzzles by ignoring reality? A theory must aim to be both tractable *and* realistic (Coase 1937). As convenient as it would be for us to suppose that modules are independently modifiable gross cognitive components, the evidence of neural reuse suggests that this is not how the brain is organized. So either the problem itself is real and the evidence of reuse must be explained away, or the assumption that no non-(massively)-modular brain could possibly evolve must be set aside. Surely the latter approach would be the more sensible. The debugging issue itself is to a large extent a symptom of looking at things a certain way. If we accept that, on some level, evolution has to involve the emergence of functionally exiguous neural parts, and view the engineering problem as being how *preexisting* parts might be combined in novel ways, concerns over debugging become far less pressing. Minimodules, in any case, are not trivial. The mind could have been (and indeed *has* been) modeled in very different ways (think connectionism/Parallel Distributed Processing, holism, etc.), and a minimodule hypothesis is quite demonstrably falsifiable (unlike, say, the system view). Minimodules also support robust predictions (like forward inference) and theory-building. The truth is that minimodules are as modular as they need to be—modular enough to solve the very real wiring problems posed by scaling circuits, and modular enough to rule competing accounts like functional holism and strict localization out of the question. The trivialization charge is a nonstarter.

What, then, of the more serious line of attack? Although there are developments of the argument in several directions, its general thrust is to make a lot of the fact that the brain implements a network. Anderson (2010, p. 249) frames the issue in these terms: "Instead of the decompose-and-localize approach to cognitive science that is advocated and exemplified by most modular accounts of the brain, neural reuse encourages 'network thinking.'" To recapitulate briefly, all networks share a number of important properties, properties that make the study of any structure that exhibits a network design far more tractable than it might otherwise be. Preeminent among these of course are nodes and edges, but a defining mark of the network approach is its focus on the global structure of *interactions* between nodes, rather than the individual nodes themselves. Thus, if the brain is a network, modularity goes awry, for even if we were to concentrate all our energies upon modules *qua* nodes (i.e., minimodules), *still* we would be missing the point—the key to networks lies not in their nodes, but in the structure of their interactions.

Such is the clear-cut statement of the challenge. Put in this form, however, it just overstates the case. First, the fact that a team of soccer players exhibits higher-order dynamics in no way obviates the importance of individual players to the game; indeed, their unique talents and skills are what drive the interactions that feature at the level of abstract topology. Second, and this is well worth remembering through all the hype, one should be no less judicious in one's use of a network analogy than in one's use of any other:

> Although the terms "network" and "connectivity" are widely used when talking about regional covariation in the human brain, it is important to keep in mind that no human data at present allow us to make inferences about brain regions forming networks in the true sense of the word. In particular, under a technical definition, two brain regions form a network if they are anatomically connected, typically via monosynaptic projections. In living humans, we rarely, if ever, can say anything conclusive about anatomical connections among brain regions. . . . [C]ollections of regions are more appropriately characterized as functional systems. (Fedorenko & Thompson-Schill 2014, p. 121)

Still, even if we were to moderate the argument in allowing for such complications, the network challenge would remain. We may for convenience describe three distinct iterations of the challenge, each more persuasive than the last, which in one way or another play upon the importance of the network context for understanding local function (inasmuch as context determines meaning). The thought here is that because minimodules appear across multiple and functionally diverse neural communities, they lack the precise degree of specialization required of modules—in view of just how tiny minimodules are, the more partnerships a given minimodule enters into, the more abstract its contribution becomes, and the dumber, simpler, and more generic it will ultimately be (Klein 2012). Price and Friston (2005, p. 268) use the example of a forefinger. Its many roles could include piano playing, typing, scratching, pinching, and feeding; yet if we had to designate its overall role, we would have to settle on something explanatorily inert: "the forefinger can only do one thing—'bend' and 'straighten.' Its role in other tasks is . . . entirely dependent on what the other fingers and thumbs are doing and what environmental context they are in." In short, "naming the specific function that a region performs (or even supposing it *has* some single specific function) involves a kind of abduction that is inherently underconstrained and uncertain" (Anderson 2014, p. 53).

Another way of framing the issue is in terms of plasticity. The more functionally versatile and unstable a brain region, the more plastic it will be (other things being equal). At the limit, ontogenetic plasticity might be so great that even sudden, swift connection changes to the neural configuration of a given brain region between alternating task demands would be possible, and functional stasis merely illusory. Up until now, neuroscientists have simply presumed that a network approach can naturally complement a modular approach—naturally, because from the minimodule perspective, modules are akin to the nodes of a coactivation graph; but the plasticity of neural regions might so undermine their functional specificity that even neuroscientists will have to give up the pretense that such node-like entities can be modules in the full-blown sense they almost always take for granted, as when they describe these regions as "functionally specific brain regions" or "regions that are selectively engaged by a particular mental process" (Fedorenko & Thompson-Schill 2014, p. 121). In the event that neuroscientists might still like to refer to these entities as modules—much in the way they conventionally use the term to describe the communities of nodes in graphs—it would be a case of terminological convenience trumping theoretical rectitude.

The weakest iteration of the challenge adds little to what has already been said, but it might note how the preponderance of afferent input pathways sustaining the brain's supramodal organization must ever so slightly color an individual module's operations as to rob it of a deep and lasting functional essence. The more functionally promiscuous a region—joining now with the visual system, now with the language system (say)—the more we can expect the neural context to impinge on the region's functional capabilities. Brain regions are by and large fairly homogeneous anyway (Buxhoeveden & Casanova 2002, p. 941). Standard histological preparations and cytoarchitectonic methods often fail to reveal anatomical differences between neighboring yet functionally distinct cortical columns. Thus an important strategy by which the brain generates difference from sameness is through the formation of different interconnection patterns among neurons and regions; indeed, often among the very *same* neurons and regions. Input channels therefore cannot be conceived as merely useful appendages to the lines of script run by distinct neural operators, as they are themselves partly constitutive of the operations performed by them. Functional promiscuity means we cannot retain a prespecified notion of function for brain regions considered in isolation of the neural contexts in which they appear.

Now it must be said that, when put like this, the argument again runs the danger of just overstating its case. For what it seems to lead to is a variety of holism. Insofar as that *is* where this line of thinking is taking us, it should be resisted, for the weight of evidence does *not* support holism, classical connectionism/PDP, or anything like it, really. With that proviso in place, the argument is a good one—functionally distinct operators with functionally distinct input criteria *can* be observed in the brain, but a moderate pitch to incorporate the effects of context would not go astray. Let us call these "*weak* context effects." Weak context effects are those that do not compromise a brain region's ability to perform a well-defined, functionally specific (albeit domain-general) operation. This is consistent with how Anderson (2010, p. 295) originally defined a *working*: "Abstractly, it is whatever single, relatively simple thing a local neural circuit *does for* or *offers to* all of the functional complexes of which the circuit is a part."

Evidence for stronger context effects is not hard to find. Let us call them "*strong* context effects." These will constitute the basis for the second and third iteration of the network challenge; but before advancing any further on this front, I should make one point clear at the outset: there is something about strong context effects—implying as they do a much higher degree of plasticity for local circuits than we have encountered so far (details to follow)—which sits uneasily with aspects of the evidence of massive redeployment presented in Chapter 3. The problem is that strong context effects are incompatible with evidence suggesting that the units of redeployment are themselves relatively fixed in nature (even after allowing for synaptogenesis, etc.). To the extent that strong context effects obtain, then, the theory of reuse requires amendment. Anderson's massive redeployment hypothesis, it will be remembered, predicts that recently evolved functions should be supported by more widely scattered regions of the brain than older ones, since it should on the whole prove easier to utilize existing circuits than to devise special-purpose circuitry afresh, "and there is little reason to suppose that the useful elements will happen to reside in neighbouring brain regions" (Anderson 2010, p. 246). Not only is the evidence that Anderson cites consistent with this prediction, it could also be taken to imply something more specific about the nature of local circuits, an implication that Anderson originally had no hesitation in drawing:

> If neural circuits could be easily put to almost any use (that is, if small neural regions were locally poly-functional, as some advocates of connectionist models suggest), then given the increased metabolic costs of maintaining long-distance connections, we would expect the circuits implementing functions to remain relatively localized. That this is not the observed pattern suggests that some functionally relevant aspect of local circuits is relatively fixed. (Anderson 2010, p. 247)

But while this is one way of interpreting the evidence, a distributed network organization might be favored by evolution for rather different reasons. As Bullmore and Sporns (2012, pp. 336–337) point out, one reason why a general principle of parsimonious cost control might be compromised in favor of far-flung neural circuits has to do with the resilience that such organization may be presumed to confer. Robustness to adverse perturbations— "[t]he degree to which the topological properties of a network are resilient to 'lesions' such as the removal of nodes or edges"—could well have more to do with the distributed structure of recently acquired capacities than with the functional fixity of local circuits. At the very least, the inference that local circuits are not especially plastic again "involves a kind of abduction that is inherently underconstrained and uncertain." Anderson himself appears to have moved on from his earlier commitment to fixed local workings, but not on account of resilience *per se*. He has lately been convinced by the evidence of strong context effects in their own right, and as a result no longer speaks of fixed local "workings," preferring instead the less rigid connotations of the term "bias" in describing the functional proclivities of local brain regions. For Anderson a cortical bias is "a set of dispositional tendencies that capture the set of inputs to which the circuit will respond and govern the form of the resulting output" (2014, p. 15)—an idea that reconciles a brain region's versatility and its overall functional durability without at the same time insinuating "that each circuit does *exactly one* specific thing" (2014, p. 16).

So what exactly, then, *are* strong context effects? I think we may usefully divide them into two broad categories. The first category—motivating the second iteration of the network challenge—would appear to suggest that small brain regions can assume radically different network states, and thereby alter their basic electrophysiological configurations, depending on the requirements of the cognitive system being used. This sort of operational, on-the-fly ontogenetic plasticity of neurocognitive resources undermines the purported functional fixity of brain regions, and hence the claim that brain regions can be modular (in the true sense of being functionally specialized). The second category—motivating the third and final iteration of the network challenge—goes even further than this by throwing into question the very legitimacy of functional decomposition as a basic strategy within the cognitive sciences. Here the thought is that "it is not as if we can identify the one fixed function of an element of the system and then worry about the effect of interactions later. Rather, the interactions are often precisely what fix local function" (Anderson 2014, p. 208). This may not at first appear to be saying much more than what was said in the first instance. In fact, its ramifications are deeply unsettling for the "decompose-and-localize" approach to cognitive science, as I shall explain more fully in a moment. Let us take these two putative categories of context effects in turn.[3]

Evidence of swift, sudden connection changes in networks begins at the single neuron level. *C. elegans* has acquired fame as the nematode for which the first neural network wiring diagram was published. It contains about 300 neurons and up to 7000 synaptic connections, simple yet complex enough to serve as a model of function-structure dynamics within higher organisms. *C. elegans* neurons perform "more than one type of circuit function, including both motor and sensory functions," and sometimes perform multiple functions within the same modality (Altun & Hall 2011). Beyond the straightforward implication here that neural reuse may be evolutionarily conserved, there are intimations of still more intriguing possibilities. "Neuromodulation" refers to a family of context effects in which it is possible for the same neuron to radically change function—and perform in just the opposite role—in response to changes in the electrophysiological, chemical, and genetic environment. One example is *C. elegans*'s olfactory neuron, AWCON, which can apparently signal both attraction and repulsion to the very same odor, depending on its neuromodulatory configuration. Another is the nocioreceptive ASH neuron, which can direct both sociality and avoidance. But neuromodulation is not restricted to *C. elegans*. Similar effects have been documented in both the pond snail and the honeybee, and there are enough instances within vertebrates to suggest that neuromodulation might be a basic evolutionary strategy for coping with scarce neural resources (Anderson 2014, p. 34). Of course, before such results could support more ambitious inferences regarding human cognition, we would need evidence of large-scale modulation in more complex organisms. In the simplest organisms, small modifications of even single synapses can have significant behavioral ramifications. In larger and more complex organisms, this is unlikely to be the case. In fact, evidence of such large-scale effects does exist, even within the human literature. Most suggestive of all is the evidence Cole et al. (2013) report for "flexible hubs" in the brain that "flexibly and rapidly shift their brain-wide functional connectivity patterns" in response to changing task demands. If brain regions really do move into different functional configurations, as distinct from being redeployed in the same state for

---

[3] I am heavily indebted to Anderson (2014) for the review that follows.

different purposes, it would imply that brain regions can be neither functionally specialized (in the sense of contributing a stable and predictable operation across their various higher-order applications) nor dissociable, both because their disruption would directly impede the operation of an equivalent system—the selfsame region considered from the standpoint of any of its alternative network states—*and* because it could well prove impossible to identify a segregatable unit of neural tissue that retained a constant form from state to state.

One upshot of this concerns theory-building. Any theory we construct that tokens a brain region subject to strong context effects will not be able to offer a fully general explanation of what that region offers to all of its networks. Even those who do not think contextualism would undermine our ability to construct powerful theories supporting strong predictions concede that we would nonetheless be in the realm of *partial* generalizations (Burnston 2016). Furthermore, part of the appeal of a theory that posits functionally specific brain regions is that it supports robust inferences: one should in principle be able to infer which brain region has been engaged simply from knowing what function is being performed. Strong context effects undermine the robustness of such inferences.

None of this entails that the brain is equipotential or has an inherently open texture (as we shall see in Chapter 6). On the contrary, overlaps between the neural implementations of cognitive tasks are frequently found to involve functional and semantic inheritance (Mather et al. 2013, pp. 109–110; see also my § 3.3), implying that brain regions have a stable set of causal features that regulates their participation in various networks. This is consistent with the finding that recently acquired skills in the human lineage, such as reading and writing, have highly uniform neural substrates across both individuals and cultures (Dehaene 2005). But when the specific point in dispute is whether the mind/brain has a modular architecture, such facts alone cannot be decisive, for then the issue is not whether brain regions have specific developmental biases, input preferences, or an underlying structural and functional integrity, but precisely the degree to which brain regions are specialized. A bias is not a specialization.

To recapitulate, so far we have considered how natural the alliance between modularity and reuse can be, and proceeded to examine various objections to this view. The objections come in two forms: weak and strong. The weak objection alleges that minimodules are trivial entities, but we saw how this claim is in fact unwarranted. The stronger objection plays on the network structure of brain organization to reveal the illusoriness of functional specialization for individual brain regions, being comparable to network nodes whose functional importance is subordinate to internodal network interactions. This stronger network challenge in turn assumes three distinct forms, one emphasizing weak context effects (which we dismissed as instructive but not fatal to modularity), and two emphasizing strong context effects. The first category of strong context effects correlates with increasing ontogenetic plasticity. The objection from these context effects really does have bite, and probably compromises the modularity of any brain region that is vulnerable to their impact. I turn now to the second category of strong context effects.

The second category raises very serious doubts over the legitimacy of componential analysis, and so by implication practically all mainstream work in the cognitive sciences. The decompose-and-localize approach to cognition assumes that the mind can be understood by analogy to a machine with working parts. Central to this approach is the belief that function can be explained in terms of "bottom-up additive contributions" rather than "top-down constraints that limit, change, or determine functional properties" (Anderson 2014, p. 308). Recent discoveries suggest this confidence may be misplaced, although quite to what extent remains unclear at this stage. The starkest illustration of these effects is offered by starburst amacrine cells (SAC) in the mammalian starburst amacrine cells (SAC) retina. These are axonless neurons with dendrites arranged radially around their cell body. "What is especially interesting about these cells is that the dendrites are *individually* differentially sensitive to motion; they release neurotransmitter only in response to motion that is congruent with the direction the dendrite points away from the cell body" (Anderson 2014, pp. 92–93). It is tempting to think of each dendrite as a component because each appears to contribute uniquely and dissociably to effects at a higher network level.

> In fact, the directional selectivity of each dendrite is due in large part to the particular blend of connections these cells have to bipolar cells and other SACs such that responses in the congruent dendrites are reinforced while responses in noncongruent dendrites are inhibited. In other words the directional selectivity of the dendrite in a given situation is due not so much to intrinsic properties of that dendrite but to global properties of the network. *Global function is not built from componential local function, but rather the reverse!* (Anderson 2014, p. 93)

While one could well think that the *entire* local network is itself a component, it should not come as a surprise if the very same dynamics "reproduce themselves at the higher level," with the functional selectivity of whatever putative higher-level component being determined again by global network properties rather than intrinsic local features. If these dynamics apply more generally to neural networks, the assumption behind componential analysis would be substantially undermined, for then no longer would components be "temporally and functionally stable subassemblies sitting on the tabletop waiting for final construction" (Anderson 2014, pp. 93–94). Instead, the "functional organization of the whole" would be logically prior to the functionally parasitic part. Put another way, *interactions between* parts would be more important than the *activity of* parts (Anderson 2014, p. 40).

Olaf Sporns has mooted similar ideas. The traditional way of thinking about circuits is in terms of "highly specific point-to-point interaction[s] among circuit elements with each link transmitting very specific information, much like an electronic or logic circuit in a computer" (Sporns 2015, p. 92). In this account, the activity of the whole circuit is "fully determined by the sum total of these specific interactions," with the corollary that "circuit function is fully decomposable . . . into neat sequences of causes and effects." This is a Laplacian model of classical mechanics, "with circuit elements exerting purely local effects." The modern approach from complexity theory and network science, however, emphasizes "that global outcomes are irreducible to simple localized causes, and that the functioning of the network *as a whole* transcends the functioning of each of its individual elements." As an example of an emergent network phenomenon, Sporns takes neural synchronization, "the coordinated firing 'in sync' of large numbers of nerve cells" (Sporns 2015, p. 93). While this phenomenon clearly depends on elemental interactions and synaptic connections, "it is not attributable to any specific causal chain of interactions in a circuit model." Rather, it is "the global outcome of many local events orchestrated by the network as a whole."

We can represent these varying degrees of modular specialization along a continuum running from A to E, each with the indicia represented in Table 5.1. Brain regions at or to the left of C, which marks the onset of weak context effects, will be sufficiently specialized to count as modular. Brain regions to the right of C, characterized by strong context effects, will not. Plasticity increases as one moves from A through D.

So *will* modularity survive evidence of neural reuse, neuromodulation, and the very strongest effects of network context? It is worth remembering

Table 5.1 A Scale of Specificity Along with Indicia of Specificity for Brain Regions

	A	B	C	D	E
			Increasing plasticity →		
	Theoretical domain specificity	**Strict domain specificity**	**Formal domain specificity**	**Neuro-modulation**	**Non-decomposition**
Indica	Minimal afferents	Few afferents	Many afferents	Many afferents	——
	Participation in a single task & composite within a single task category	Participation in various tasks & composites within a single task category	Participation in various tasks & composites within various task categories	Participation in various tasks & composites within various task categories	——
	Nonreuse	Nonreuse	Reuse	Reuse	——
	No context effects	Negligible context effects	Weak context effects	Dynamic local network states	Local function fixed by global properties
	Functional specialization	Functional specialization	Functional specialization	Functional differentiation	Functional differentiation
Possible examples	Probably none–a theoretical postulate only	Neural element common & exclusive to reading, writing & speaking; e.g., the neural basis of subjacency/*wh* movement	Extrastriate body area; Broca's area	Flexible "hubs" in the brain reported by Cole et al. (2013)	Starburst amacrine cells; synchronization

that at this stage the case for the very strongest of context effects is still speculative. Russell Poldrack, for his part—whose laboratory work in this space has been pioneering (e.g., Poldrack et al. 2009)—is convinced that cognitive systems will bottom out in low-level, domain-general and functionally specific computational operations bearing a one-to-one relationship to specific cortical sites. On the other hand, if neuromodulatory and context effects are indeed as pervasive and game-changing as some people seem to think (e.g., Bach-y-Rita 2004), perhaps only a few scattered islands of modularity are all we can reasonably hope for (Prinz 2006). It is true that employing current techniques it is not actually possible to assign brain regions to definite locations on a continuum, so we cannot know for sure that only a few brain regions will cluster towards the specialist end (e.g., A through C, as mentioned). But evidence for the existence, power, and ubiquity of context effects can only proliferate at this point, one would think. (Incidentally—taking up a point I raised in § 4.3—if the "modules" reaching into central cognition turn out to have type D characteristics, central cognition will be *pro tanto* nonmodular after all. See § 7.2.2 for further discussion.)

It is worth mentioning that the picture here is consistent with the emerging consensus around the neocortical column we met in § 4.3 (Rockland 2010; see da Costa & Martin 2010 for a historical review). Rockland takes five defining features of the column and argues that these are too rigid to do justice to the complexity of cortical organization. For instance, it is supposed that columns are solid structures, but this is not quite true, since they have a heterogeneous substructure that "correlates with reports of locally heterogeneous response properties," very much as reuse predicts (Rockland 2010, p. 3). Their anatomy is therefore messy rather than solid. Columns also form part of widely distributed networks at several levels (again, much as reuse predicts), and for that matter are not even obligatory to cortex: for instance "comparative anatomy provides many examples of cortex apparently without anatomical columns or dramatically modified columns," such as in whales and dolphins, whose insular cortices have cellular modules concentrated in layer II, and the giraffe, whose occipital cortex has modules concentrated in the same layer (Rockland 2010, p. 7).

I think it is fair to say, then, that while most of the cortex undoubtedly consists of module-like elements, probably only a few of these will in the end prove to be modular in the robust sense we require. The full implications of network thinking for componential analysis in particular have not sunk in, even though they promise to overturn our conception of local function almost completely. It goes without saying, of course, that to the extent that modules *do* exist, it will be as functionally exiguous and promiscuous brain regions. The days of classical modularity are well and truly over.

5.2 Can Composite Systems Be Dissociable?

Up to this point in the discussion, I have simply assumed that a cognitive system consisting of shared domain-general parts cannot *ipso facto* be separately modifiable. Some, however, have maintained that neural overlaps need *not* undermine the functional independence of high-level cognitive functions (Carruthers 2006, pp. 23–24). This is just to raise the possibility that high-level cognitive functions could persist as *functional* modules (as distinct from *anatomical* modules).

It is undoubtedly true that, of any two cognitive systems considered in isolation, the extent of neural overlap may be only partial, or even negligible. This would render the two systems dissociable vis-à-vis each other to the extent that a modification not affecting shared components would disrupt or improve the affected system independently. But this kind of dissociability—the dissociability of a cognitive system relative to another—comes cheap. Imagine that function A is implemented in the left lateral hemisphere, while function B is implemented in the right lateral hemisphere. The two functions are spatially far apart, and (let us say) may be sufficiently far apart that interventions affecting A will not directly affect B. In this case, relative to each other, it will be true that functions A and B are dissociable (indeed, doubly so). But this is compatible with function A's being fully nondissociable relative to functions C and D (in the left cerebral hemisphere), and function B's being fully nondissociable relative to functions E and F (in the right cerebral hemisphere). In short, any two cognitive systems that are functionally independent vis-à-vis each other may yet lack functional independence vis-à-vis any number of other cognitive systems. Taking high-level cognitive systems two at a time is an easy way to demonstrate functional independence. But in the brain, functions do not come two at a time.

A stronger consideration that argues in favor of functional independence for overlapping systems is this:

at the limit, two modules could share *all* of their processing parts while still remaining dissociable and separately modifiable. For the differences might lie entirely in the patterns of connectivity among the parts, in such a way that those connections could be separately disrupted or improved. (Ritchie & Carruthers 2010, p. 289)

If—going back to functions A and B as discussed here—it could be shown that any of the connection pathways utilized in function A are exclusive to A, such that no other cognitive system makes use of them, it would seem that, to the extent that A's pathways are unique to A, A would to that extent be functionally independent. (If the same could be said for the pathways utilized in function B, B would likewise—and to that extent—be functionally independent.)

While the consideration is a powerful one, its standing can only be settled empirically. And the evidence we have gives us no reason to suspect that reuse is limited to columns. Neurons, too, can be reused, which—as far as we know—means that *all* of their parts (cell bodies, dendrites, axons, and, importantly, synapses) will be extensively reused throughout the brain. Thus, once the true scale of reuse dawns, the claim that high-level cognitive functions may persist as functional modules appears less convincing.

5.3 Modular Notation

Perhaps the single most important upshot of the discussion so far has been that modularity can no longer serve in the role of marking a traditional cognitive ontology. We have seen how modules (really "minimodules") are both structurally and functionally exiguous, and so nowhere up to the job of supporting functions as complex as language (or even vision!) taken by themselves. In this section, I shall provide a simple notation to express at a glance the essential features of the new perspective I am advocating. It will serve as a convenient shorthand with which to convey some of the more important points relating to the search for a language module in Chapter 7. Thus, let us take modules to be defined by the set

$$\{M_1, M_2, M_3 \ldots M_n\}$$

where M_1, M_2, etc., are modules. Modules are really small networks of neurons, and can for convenience be labelled "M-networks" (to distinguish them from the many higher-level networks in which modules participate in turn). Thus a module can be defined by the set

$$\{N_1, N_2, N_3 \ldots N_n\}$$

where N_1, N_2, etc., are neurons, so that a given module M_a will comprise a set of neurons

$$M_a : \{N_a, N_b, N_c, \ldots\}$$

An M-network is (or resembles) the structure that neuroscience variously terms a "module," "column," or "elementary processing unit," and that Bergeron (2007, 2008), and Anderson (2010, 2015) originally, called a "working." It consists of around 6000 neurons or 60–80 minicolumns, each minicolumn consisting of between 80 and 100 neurons (Buxhoeveden & Casanova 2002, p. 935). The higher-level functional composites in which modules participate are themselves networks (call them "C-networks"). We can take C-networks to be defined by the set

$$\{C_1, C_2, C_3 \ldots C_n\}$$

where C_1, C_2, etc., are C-networks, so that a given C-network C_a will be a set of M-networks

$$C_a : \{M_a, M_b, M_c, \ldots\}$$

I take M-networks and C-networks to be the central *explananda* of cognitive neuroscience. Given the rather drab prognosis with which I concluded § 5.1, we should expect to find only a smattering of real M-networks in the cortex, and that many of the structures that neuroscientists have identified as modules have been technically misdescribed.

Over the years, the attention of psychologists and cognitive scientists has quite understandably been lavished upon the functional taxonomies that C-networks serve to implement. But, as I have suggested several times already, the same scientists often thought they were dealing with something having the structural characteristics of an M-network. This was most unfortunate, and its ill-effects have by no means been eradicated. Such misconceptions necessarily inform both the design and the interpretation of scientific experiments. The debate about whether the fusiform gyrus is specialized for faces, to take only one example, "has unfolded in the context of the shared belief that the ventral visual areas are specialized for recognizing some classes of objects," a belief that is no longer tenable, pending further notice (Gold & Roskies 2008, p. 354).

To sum up, then, there are at least two networks of interest as far as the modularity of mind is concerned: the network of neurons that constitutes a node/M-network, and the network of nodes that constitutes a composite of nodes/C-network. The former is what has come to be regarded as a module in mainstream neuroscience, while the latter is regarded as a module among those working with graphs in network neuroscience. This latter notion, as we saw, has obvious affinities with the mental modules familiar to cognitive scientists, psychologists, and philosophers, since it seems to track quite readily the ontologies of traditional psychology (language, vision, face-recognition, etc.). One cannot, however, assume that mental modules (Fodorian or otherwise) can be reduced smoothly to the communities of nodes that are studied extensively in graph theory (Anderson 2010, p. 303, 2014, p. 42). Quite apart from other differences, the classic Fodorian module is an anatomical module, and hence functionally dissociable and localized in relatively segregated neural tissue. This is not the case of graph-theoretic (network neuroscience) modules, as I explained earlier. If Fodor's module has any legitimate successor at all, then, it must be something with relative stimulus specificity and informational autonomy—something with the functional characteristics of an M-network.

5.4 Summary

In Chapter 4, I argued that we ought to regard dissociability as the *sine qua non* of modularity. As for what in the brain interestingly meets this standard, the only likely candidate will be something resembling a cortical column. But this is not guaranteed. The effects of the neural network context may so compromise a region's ability to maintain a set of stable input–output relations that it cannot be considered a genuine module.

6

Are Modules Innate?

6.1 Preliminary Remarks

Asking whether modules are innate is problematic for at least three reasons. First, the conclusion of the previous chapter suggests that the subject of the question is not appropriate: we would do better to ask whether *brain regions* are innate. Second, there is the rather thorny issue of what one actually means by "innate." Third, the question assumes that a *general* answer can be given, when it is unlikely that all (or even most) brain structures will have the same developmental story to tell: "there will be cases and cases" (Mameli & Papineau 2006, p. 564). This last concern can be alleviated by concentrating the weight of one's empirical attention on a particular module, if not by having regard to as much brain-wide evidence as possible. Chapter 2 was my attempt to incorporate a wide survey of the evidence of neuroplasticity—with as many caveats and limiting clauses as its interpretation reasonably warrants—while Chapter 7 is my attempt to home in on one particular system (namely, language). In the present chapter, I aim to build on the interpretation of neuroplasticity that I began in Chapter 2.

This still of course leaves us with the problem of having to define what we mean by "innateness," a far from trivial matter (Griffiths 2002; Mameli & Bateson 2006; Bateson & Mameli 2007; Mameli & Bateson 2011). The trouble is that the term is as ambiguous as it is entrenched, and some have wondered whether it can perform a useful function in the sciences at all. With so large a variety of distinct notions lying beneath the surface, it becomes very easy to commit fallacies of ambiguity (Griffiths et al. 2009). One might, for example, infer that a trait is species-typical by virtue of its being the product of natural selection, or developmentally fixed by virtue of its being species-typical (O'Neill 2015). In the result Griffiths (2002) recommends having done with the term altogether, and suggests that scientists should specify explicitly what they mean on any given occasion. I do not take an "eliminativist" stance

The Adaptable Mind. John Zerilli, Oxford University Press (2021). © Oxford University Press.
DOI: 10.1093/oso/9780190067885.003.0006

myself, but, along with Griffiths, do think it absolutely essential to make explicit the sense in which the term is being used. Following O'Neill (2015), what I have in mind is *insensitivity relative to some specific set of environmental variations.* This is the idea of developmental robustness or environmental canalization, broadly speaking (Ariew 1996, 1999, 2007; Mameli & Bateson 2006; O'Neill 2015), except that it is explicitly relativized to specific environmental factors (Bateson & Mameli 2007, p. 823).[1] After all, no trait is developmentally robust in an absolute sense, yet the claim is frequently made without specifying the environmental factors with respect to which the trait is supposed to be robust. For the most part this is not a problem, since it is usually clear in a given context which environmental factors are relevant (O'Neill 2015, p. 212). Still, it is important to bear in mind that a trait's invariance (or otherwise) is always relative. In the present context, we are concerned with the innateness of modules—iterated cortical structures with distinctive columnar and laminar patterns of organization. It should by now be clear that modules are not insensitive with respect to such experiences as learning, injury, and sensory deprivation, regardless of how young or mature the organism happens to be. The extent of both intramodal and crossmodal plasticity, as well as evidence for the extensive rewiring of latent supramodal connection channels, does much to discredit the traditional nativist assumption of "hardwired" cognitive capacities with rigid developmental schedules (Marcus 2004).

Yet this cannot be the full story. For one thing, sensitivity with respect to a particular set of environmental factors does not entail sensitivity with respect to others; and in the absence of factors to which a trait *is* sensitive, its development might well be considered robust. For instance, when developmental biologists speak of "activity-independent" cell differentiation, which results in cortical areas' acquiring fixed structural characteristics *in utero*, they can be taken to imply that at least some aspects of modular development are insensitive relative to certain factors, although obviously not with respect to the factors that can be expected to become influential at a later stage of

---

[1] I say *broadly* speaking because *strictly* speaking, canalization results in a "buffered" developmental pathway in which insensitivity with respect to some environmental factor is the result of a specific mechanism or evolutionary adaptation geared to that end (e.g., Waddington 1953, 1955). But insensitivity *simpliciter* can be the result of an environmental factor's having no causal influence on a trait at all. A fly's wing pattern could be insensitive to certain pesticides without having been buffered against them by natural selection; e.g., because the pesticides concerned do not interact causally with the fly's development in any way (O'Neill 2015).

development; i.e., during postnatal "activity-dependent" cell differentiation (Saitoe & Tully 2001, p. 193; Kolb et al. 2001, p. 225; Sanes & Jessell 2013, p. 1259).[2] Furthermore, sensitivity admits of degrees (Collins 2005). Granted that cortical development is robust in certain respects, *how* robust is an important question in each case. Thus there are really two senses in which we can speak of invariance as being a matter of degree: along one dimension, we can say that the more factors with respect to which a trait is robust, the more invariant it will be; while along a second dimension, the more a trait is robust to variation in any *single* factor, the more invariant it will be (Griffiths & Machery 2008, p. 399). One may therefore legitimately inquire as to whether cell differentiation results in a stereotyped but essentially crude pattern of synaptic connections and brain regions before birth, or whether it results in more robust operations that limit and constrain the functions these regions can later take on. There is scope for genuine disagreement here between those who think there is a lot of prewiring, combined with some inevitable rewiring during development (Marcus 2004), and those who think there is comparatively little prewiring, with a lot of rewiring during development and later life (see the discussion by Mameli & Papineau 2006, pp. 563–564).

In this chapter, I shall argue that the evidence of neuroplasticity supports neither a traditional nativist nor yet a strictly antinativist interpretation of development. Rather, we seem to be confronting a phenomenon that falls somewhere midway between the two extremes of developmental hardwiring and original equipotentiality. While the extent of the neuroplastic responses we considered in Chapter 2 is undoubtedly impressive, and sometimes vast, a closer look at these cases suggests that the pattern of responses is constrained. For all their plasticity, brain modules and regions appear to be significantly robust in the presence of such environmental variables as learning, injury, and sensory deprivation. More precisely, the changes that do occur are exactly what one would expect to find under the assumption that cortical regions have robust processing capabilities and clear input preferences (what I earlier described as a "bias"). This is not a traditional nativist picture, to be sure, but neither is it antinativist. (Warning: the evidence to follow is circumstantial, the argumentation non-demonstrative and abductive. In the realm of cognition, however, we frequently find ourselves with little else to go on.)

---

[2] Moreover, a trait's sensitivity with respect to a set of experiences at one stage of development does not preclude its being insensitive with respect to the same experiences at an earlier stage (Kolb et al. 2001, pp. 223, 225; Mameli & Bateson 2006, p. 169; see also my § 2.3).

6.2 Implications of Neuroplasticity

Of all the instances of cortical map plasticity we reviewed in Chapter 2, undoubtedly the most impressive involve crossmodal changes in which brain regions deprived of their typical inputs come to subserve alternative uses. One example I mentioned there concerned early-blind Braille readers whose visual cortex appears to be functionally important for Braille character identification, suggesting a functional contribution of the reorganized occipital cortices during complex tactile discrimination tasks (Sadato et al. 1996). Moreover, when repetitive transcranial magnetic stimulation (rTMS) is used to impair the functioning of the occipital cortex, blind subjects appear to have difficulty performing embossed-character recognition, while sighted control subjects do not, again pointing up the functional significance of early-blind occipital cortices during tactile discrimination (Cohen et al. 1997). Probably the most famous case of crossmodal plasticity is that of the rewired ferrets whose visual cortex was induced to project into auditory cortex after their retinal nerves were rerouted so that, instead of feeding into primary visual cortex, they fed into primary auditory cortex via the auditory thalamus (Sharma et al. 2000; Melchner et al. 2000). The manipulation resulted in ferret auditory cortex's taking on features typical of occipital cortex, such as columnar orientation and stimulus selectivity. Besides these cases, language studies suggest that this sort of plasticity is not confined to sensory-motor cortices alone, as the case of EB discussed in Chapter 2 illustrates very well.

While these results seem quite dramatic, nevertheless, some aspects of the evidence do not fit well with the idea of the brain as open-endedly malleable. In fact, rather than supporting the case for plasticity *tout court*, these results argue the case for what Laurence and Margolis (2015) call "constrained plasticity." Take the ferret case. The clear suggestion here is that auditory cortex came to resemble the processing structures typically associated with occipital cortex. And indeed, to *some* extent, this is what seems to have happened. But in fact, primary occipital cortex is a complicated structure, "connected to a large number of distinct brain regions that support further specific types of visual processing, including computations responsible for downstream representations of location, direction of motion, speed, shape, and so on" (Laurence & Margolis 2015, p. 127). And there is no evidence that any of this complex processing structure was reproduced, for "the overall wiring of the ferrets' auditory cortex was largely unchanged." One interpretation of why a "largely unchanged" auditory cortex was able to process visual inputs is consonant with the theory of supramodal organization (and Pascual-Leone and Hamilton's metamodal hypothesis). Recall that this theory posits a large number of intrinsically stable neural operators that are more or less suited to processing specific types of input, but are at the same time metamodal in that they receive inputs from many domains (i.e., they are really domain-general, or formally domain-specific). From this perspective, we would naturally expect there to be something about visual and auditory stimuli that makes them ideal for a neural operator whose processing disposition makes it suited to process one or the other of these specific types of input. Bregman and Pinker (1978) long ago postulated high-level analogies in computations that involve auditory and visual stimuli (e.g., different pitches are analogous to different locations, pronounced changes of pitch are analogous to sudden changes in the direction of motion, etc.). If such analogies between hearing and vision hold, it would suggest—consistently with the metamodal hypothesis—that auditory cortex did not really *need* to change when it began to receive inputs from a domain to which its processing capabilities were already well suited. As Laurence and Margolis interpret the ferret case:

> even though the rewiring experiments show that the auditory cortex can be recruited for a certain amount of visual processing, this is because the auditory cortex and the visual cortex overlap in the types of computations they naturally support. Far from being a model case of the environment instructing an equipotential cortex, [the ferret] rewiring experiments illustrate the way in which cortical structure and function remain largely unchanged even in the extreme case of input coming from a different sensory system. (2015, p. 128)

Next, consider the case of EB from Chapter 2. EB recovered most of his language skills two years after undergoing a left hemispherectomy at the age of two and a half and tested as largely normal with respect to language at age 14, albeit with his language faculty now subserved by regions in his right cerebral hemisphere. Surely this argues for an almost equipotential cortex early in development, if anything does? Not quite. The fMRI evidence showed that the pattern of activation in his right hemisphere was almost isomorphic to that of the left hemisphere in normal control subjects, revealing a definite and predictable cortical pattern. Language did not arbitrarily migrate to a new location: it moved to the very site in the right hemisphere whose structural features most nearly resemble those of the left hemisphere's language circuits. A truly equipotential brain would presumably reconfigure cortical sites selected on a far more *ad hoc* basis. The most important take-home message here, then, is not that the brain is open-endedly plastic, but rather that "the brain's two hemispheres incorporate a large measure of potential redundancy of function that can be exploited at certain stages of development" (Laurence & Margolis 2015, p. 126; see also my § 7.5).

These cases are only a beginning. By far the most significant evidence for constrained plasticity and the robust development of brain regions comes from studies revealing the brain's latent supramodal organization. A flavor of this evidence was given in § 2.4.3, but it is instructive to consider a few more examples to drive the point home. It will be remembered that evidence of supramodal organization first came from studies of the two major visual processing streams; i.e., the dorsal ("action") path for space and motion discrimination, and the ventral ("categorization") path for object and shape recognition. What these studies suggest is that this dual stream processing structure persists with the same functional role and structural characteristics in both early and congenitally blind and sighted subjects. That is to say, even total and protracted visual input inhibition—from the very earliest developmental stages onwards—appears to have few if any adverse effects on the development of typical visual processing structures in humans. To repeat the conclusion one researcher drew from the case we examined in Chapter 2, "despite the vast plasticity of the cortex to process other sensory inputs," these findings suggest "retention of functional specialization in this same region" (Striem-Amit & Amedi 2014, p. 4). The dorsal and ventral processing streams appear to be modular, developmentally constrained, and functionally preserved despite complete early and congenital visual impairment.

In one study (Renier et al. 2010), early-blind subjects were presented with paired auditory stimuli that differed either in type (in this case, different piano chords) or locality.[3] The task required subjects to indicate whether the pairings were of the same type or emanated from the same location. Subjects exhibited differential activation in a region of the dorsal visual stream—specifically, the area rostral to the right middle occipital gyrus (MOG)—when engaged in the auditory spatial location task relative to the sound-type identification task. Similar results were obtained on an analogous tactile discrimination task using the same subjects. So while the MOG is clearly plastic, in that early-blind individuals recruit this area more intensively for auditory

---

[3] The examples in this paragraph and the next are drawn from Laurence and Margolis (2015).

and tactile discrimination tasks than do sighted individuals, its plasticity reveals it to be functionally constrained and structurally preserved. It is classically supramodal in that it continues to perform a fixed computation despite receiving different sensory input. Other studies attest to the persistence of the spatial location function of the dorsal visual stream. Consider the posterior parietal cortex (PPC), implicated in the spatial representations that guide action. In healthy sighted subjects, caudal subregions play a relatively larger role in reaching and grasping than do rostral subregions, which are primarily engaged in the planning and execution of action. Lingnau et al. (2014) showed that the same response gradient occurs in the congenitally blind, concluding that "neural plasticity acts within a relatively rigid framework of predetermined functional specialization" (2014, p. 547). Other studies evidence preservation of the direction representation function of the dorsal visual stream, as judged by performance of congenitally blind subjects on analogous auditory discrimination tasks (Wolbers et al. 2011), as well as functions in the ventral visual stream in both congenitally blind and blindfolded sighted subjects (as we saw in Chapter 2) (Striem-Amit et al. 2012; Striem-Amit & Amedi 2014). Laurence and Margolis conclude their review of this evidence in the following way:

> it would appear that the large-scale functional architecture of the visual cortex—the division of labor between the dorsal and ventral streams—develops in much the same way, and with the same functions being performed in various subregions of these streams, with or without visual experience. (2015, p. 133)

And of course all of this evidence once again testifies to the supramodal organization of the brain, and Pascual-Leone and Hamilton's metamodal hypothesis in particular, since it is consistent with a brain that is composed of a number of "distinct computational systems whose functions are established independently of their sensory input" (Laurence & Margolis 2015, p. 428) and in which "multimodal sensory inputs feed into all cortical regions" (Pascual-Leone & Hamilton 2001, p. 432), even though the operations of a given region will dictate certain preferences. The metamodal hypothesis predicts that "when the preferred input is unavailable, the brain switches to the next best fit" (Laurence & Margolis 2015, p. 428) such that a region's underlying computational structure and profile need undergo no truly radical alteration in the face of new processing inputs—in the standard case, it will perform in much the same way it always did, albeit on a new set of afferents. In this view, even many dramatic instances of crossmodal plasticity, where the equipotential nature of the cortex seems to be its most obvious feature, need involve little more than a straightforward remodeling of supramodal connection channels (Pascual-Leone & Hamilton 2001, p. 443).

One final study is especially worth mentioning for the illumination it provides on the precise extent to which predefined cortical functionality is developmentally robust. A group of mice whose brains were genetically modified so that they were incapable of synaptic transmission, and therefore incapable of releasing any neurotransmitters at all, were compared to normal control littermates. Mice in whom the potential for all synaptic transmission has been inhibited in this way have effectively no potential for learning or indeed any *activity-dependent* cell differentiation. Verhage et al. (2000) reported that, at least prior to birth, the two brain types were assembled correctly, and were in fact essentially similar. As they state their own findings:

> Neuronal proliferation, migration and differentiation into specific brain areas were unaffected. At [embryonic day 12], brains from null mutant and control littermates were morphologically indistinguishable. . . . At birth, late-forming brain areas such as the neocortex appeared identical in null mutant and control littermates, including a distinctive segregation of neurons into cortical layers. . . . Furthermore, fiber pathways were targeted correctly in null mutants. (2000, p. 866)

This means activity-*independent* changes are robust enough to withstand severe synaptic privation, and "that many features of even the fine-grained structure of the brain can develop without any sensory input or feedback" (Laurence & Margolis 2015, p. 130).

Notice, incidentally, just what this sort of neuroconstructivist nativism implies: that while there is a certain (and relative) sense in which M-networks and other functionally significant brain regions are developmentally robust, the same cannot be said for higher-level cognitive functions. There is a weak sense, of course, in which the innateness of M-networks translates to the innateness of higher-level/gross functional composites, which are innate insofar as the parts used in assembling them are innate. But this claim is different from the claim that such higher-level composites are innate *as organized* (Jusczyk & Cohen 1985). If the "derived" innateness of a functional composite were sufficient for its being considered innate as an organized ensemble, all complex cognitive functions would be innate by default, which is plainly absurd. I shall revisit this matter in Chapter 7 (see pp. 120–121).

Before I leave this chapter, it will be useful to delineate once again the relationship between neuroplasticity (*qua* Hebbian learning) and neural reuse, for there is a good deal of complementarity on offer here that is easy to miss amid the detail of specific cases. The supramodally organized brain in effect constitutes the architectural foundation upon which Hebbian synaptic mechanisms operate. That is to say, Hebbian plasticity presupposes reuse, inasmuch as it consists in the strengthening (or weakening) of *existing* supramodal connection channels. Synaptic pruning, synaptogenesis, and other forms of interneural transmission can no doubt account for the more drastic examples of plastic change and post-pathological recovery we examined in Chapter 2 (yielding "a change in use from a change in working," in the language of Chapter 3), perhaps joining a suite of mechanisms that could account for the very youngest cortico-cortical pathways established in the developing brain (in effect supplying us with a supramodal architectural foundation).[4] But Hebbian mechanisms remain an important part of the story of how patterns of neural reuse are regularly refined and remodeled in the course of normal development, learning, and recovery after injury (yielding "a change in use *without* a change in working," as we saw in Chapter 3).

6.3 Summary

The brain's plasticity is definitely constrained. While plasticity is an intrinsic and crucial feature of the nervous system, it is important to emphasize that the brain is not open-endedly plastic. Furthermore, a brain region can be innate in a relatively strong sense and yet fail to reach the threshold characteristics of a genuine module. A bias, after all, is not a specialization.

---

[4] Anderson (2014) hypothesizes such a suite of mechanisms under the label "search." I return to this idea in Chapter 7, with a twist of my own.

7

The Language Module Reconsidered

7.1 Preliminary Remarks

The contention that language is domain-dedicated and innate is as much a claim about cerebral organization as it is about function. My aim in this chapter is to extend the framework provided so far by offering an account of how language could be implemented in brains in a way that honors its autonomy, developmental robustness, and connection to other domains. Any examination of the relevant literature will quickly dispel the illusion that there can be certainty in a field like this, at least for the present. But there is more than enough evidence, I think, to make the prospects of some proposals doubtful enough to warrant serious skepticism—in particular, the claim that language is subserved by hardwired and dedicated neural circuitry—and enough evidence, too, to provide the basis for a sensible if only tentative conception of neurolinguistic organization. Because all such proposals to date (no matter how vigorously and at times dogmatically defended) have been advanced in a spirit of scientific speculation, my own, of course, will be no different. I intend my thoughts on the subject to count as one further effort in the ongoing attempt to render plausible how something with the particular characteristics of language could be implemented in a domain-general architecture. The need for such a project to succeed has become urgent, in my view, precisely because the alternative is too much at odds with what we do know about the brain. Short of compelling reasons to the contrary, a theory of cognitive architecture should strive to be consistent with as much of the hard evidence that we have at our disposal, be it neural, psycholinguistic, developmental, evolutionary, or computational. But domain-specific accounts of the functional architecture of language can no longer assert that they meet this desideratum.

I should note that, while the framework of reuse I have adopted in the book so far will continue to do work for me in the present context, I shall at this juncture have to part company with Anderson and other proponents

The Adaptable Mind. John Zerilli, Oxford University Press (2021). © Oxford University Press.
DOI: 10.1093/oso/9780190067885.003.0007

of reuse. After much reflection, I have come around to the view that neural redundancy should be assigned a much more prominent role in theories of cognitive architecture than many proponents of neural reuse seem willing to contemplate. It strikes me that, in view of how simple and powerful the principle is, it is a wonder that more has not been made of it in debates concerning the modularity of mind. In my view, this is a significant omission, although happily one that, if remedied, can go a long way towards reconciling the evidence of linguistic modularization and neural reuse. I introduce what I call "the Redundancy Model" in § 7.5.

The chapter proceeds as follows. First up, we need to get a little more clarity on the very idea of a "language module." What are we looking for? What does it mean to say that language is modular, or represents a cognitive specialization? Any answer presupposes some conception of the language domain as a psychological phenomenon, as well as some conception of specialization at the level of implementation. Regarding the second issue, I should think I have already said enough, so even though I rehearse a couple of competing conceptions later in this chapter, I do not intend to modify the position that has sustained the investigation thus far. Regarding the first issue, however, I have so far said very little. The two most influential conceptions of the language domain are those associated with the linguist Noam Chomsky and the philosopher Jerry Fodor. While it would not be wrong to see these two thinkers as belonging to the same broad school of thought, their conceptions of language—of what it is we should be looking for *within* a language module—are very different. The evidence I adduce raises problems for any defender of linguistic modularity, no matter where they fall on the Chomsky–Fodor spectrum.

Next, I survey evidence of the extensive reuse of language circuits across various cognitive domains. This evidence speaks loudest against the conventional wisdom concerning a dedicated faculty of language, and converging evidence from other sources corroborates this view. At the level of implementation, then, it seems language is *not* special vis-à-vis other cognitive domains. But this then raises the old question about the robustness of language acquisition in children. The evidence of a "poverty of stimulus" continues to baffle many researches across the cognitive sciences, and it is the main motivation behind the persistent and (still) pervasive conviction that language must after all be special. The section following therefore addresses the poverty-of-stimulus issue, but in a spirit rather different from that which has been typical in discussions of linguistic nativism. Instead of throwing mud at the poverty-of-stimulus argument in the hope that some of it sticks (some of it certainly does, but enough people have thrown it for me to feel justified in moving on), I consider how a fairly robust species trait like language can be supported within a thoroughly domain-general architecture. To cap off, I parlay everything canvassed in the discussion up to this point into a general outline of how language could be implemented in the brain so that its autonomy and apparent dissociability may be fully accommodated alongside the evidence of its reuse and relative ontogenetic robustness. Here the Redundancy Model comes to the fore.

As I pointed out earlier, the principle of neural redundancy has not featured prominently in debates concerning the modularity of mind. The basic idea here is that, no doubt for good evolutionary reasons, the brain incorporates a large measure of redundancy of function. We do not seem to exhibit what has been referred to as modular *solitarity*—a single token module for each type of module that we possess.[1] Instead, we come equipped with very many tokens of the same type of module or brain region densely packed into contiguous regions of cortex. I submit that this fact can account for a lot of what we see when we examine the evidence of cognitive dissociations. More importantly, it can provide an elegant and simple solution to the engineering problem posed by the fact that many of our psychological faculties (speech, problem-solving, playing musical instruments, etc.) seem to require multiple simultaneous use of the same sorts of underlying cognitive mechanisms (the *time-sharing* problem). There is also evidence that quite often the same sorts of mechanisms are recruited for deliberative "central system" functions on one hand and fast/automatic or "peripheral" functions on the other. This is puzzling because the degree of cognitive impenetrability on display plausibly calls for segregated circuitry (the *encapsulation* problem). Redundancy naturally explains the data here, too. In fact, for all we know, redundancy might help explain many other quirks of cognition that have so far proved elusive within classical cognitive science paradigms, hostile as they often have been to implementational considerations. The same solution could suffice to solve several problems.

A good chunk of the evidence of reuse comes from neuroimaging data, but as I already indicated in Chapter 3, concerns over the spatial resolution of current imaging technologies have been played as a possible trump card

---

[1] The term "solitarity" is a neologism. See § 7.5.

against the idea of the *literal* reuse of neural circuits. While neuroimaging evidence is not the only evidence on point, and converging biobehavioral evidence also points to the extensive redeployment of the self-same neural technology, still, the likelihood of *some* cognitive mechanisms running in parallel and in close spatial proximity cannot be discounted, and indeed seems rather high given what we know of the iterative, tessellated, and almost lattice-like arrangement of modules in the cortex. The Redundancy Model beautifully supplements and extends the reuse picture in a way that is completely consistent with the neuroimaging data, faithful to the core principle of reuse, and compatible with the apparent modularization of technical and acquired skills in ontogeny. As I shall explain—and in keeping with the constrained plasticity model I presented in Chapter 6—it chimes with the motto that some modules are "made, not born," but without crude assumptions about the nearly limitless malleability of cortical tissue. In sum, it gives us just what we need to explain a (mini)modular yet fully domain-general cognitive system within a sensible and neurobiologically informed framework of explanation.

7.2 Defining a Language Module

7.2.1 The meaning of linguistic specialization

There is a clear consensus in modern neuroscience that language is mediated by "defined sets of circuits" (Fisher 2015, pp. 150–151). The main debate over these circuits concerns whether they are specific to language (Chomsky 2005, 2010). In Chapter 3, I raised the possibility that, despite extensive evidence of the reuse of neural circuits and what appears to be the deeply interpenetrative nature of mental functions, some small component or set of components is rarely coopted outside the language domain. Such a component (or set thereof) would be strictly specialized for language in its being recruited predominantly, perhaps even exclusively, for linguistic purposes. By way of example, I mentioned the possibility of a neuron or restricted set of neurons' being dedicated to conjugating the verb "to be" and having no nonlinguistic functions at all (other examples are discussed in § 7.2.3). I said that this component might aptly be described as a language "module." The debate over the specialization of linguistic function, then, can be understood as a debate concerning the existence of such modules (Fedorenko & Thompson-Schill 2014). It is an important question in its own right, of course (cf. Fitch

2010), but it carries further implications for other inquiries into the human cognitive system, as well as for the evolution of language. Among the various alternative ways of construing the issue (as to which, see later in this chapter), this is the understanding with which I shall proceed here. Let me, however, define the problem more precisely before I turn to address it directly in the following sections of this chapter.

So far, we have seen how the evidence of neural reuse strongly suggests that the only dissociable unit we are likely to encounter in the brain will be one that resembles the neuroscientific notion of a module. The neuroscientific module is sometimes called a "brain module" or "cortical module" (Mountcastle 1978, 1997; Pascual-Leone & Hamilton 2001; Gold & Roskies 2008; Rowland & Moser 2014; Zador 2015); at other times a "cortical column" or "columnar module" (Mountcastle 1978, 1997; Buxhoeveden & Casanova 2002; Amaral & Strick 2013; Zador 2015), at still other times an "elementary processing unit" (Kandel & Hudspeth 2013), or simply an "operator" (Pascual-Leone & Hamilton 2001; Pascual-Leone et al. 2005). It corresponds (very roughly) with the node of a neural coactivation graph and is known to perform only exiguous subfunctions such as aspects of edge detection or depth discrimination—certainly nothing as high-order as language acquisition or norm acquisition *per se*. High-order complex functions are instead enabled by neural ensembles or composites, which are just so many arrangements of these low-level neural modules, often highly distributed across the cortex (therefore not localized, contrary to much traditional speculation). But we also saw that, owing to the effects of the many different neural contexts in which modules appear (namely, the functional assemblies instantiating high-level complex functions), it is not clear that such units will always possess the requisite degree of specialization required to sustain their modularity: in many cases, the label "module" may actually be a misnomer. The true extent of modularity in the cortex—even with the benefit of a neuroscientifically informed conception to hand—is very much an open question. As a way of coming to grips with this issue, in Chapter 5 I provided a scale of specificity for brain regions that makes their indicia of specificity explicit. Situating the question of the modularity of language within this framework sharpens the issue considerably and shows up useful points of contrast with alternative construals. Varying degrees of modular specialization can be represented along a continuum running from A to E, each with the indicia as specified in Table 5.1 (p. 79). Brain regions at or to the left of C, which marks the onset of weak context effects, will be sufficiently specialized to count as modular. Brain regions to the right of C, characterized by strong context effects, will not. Again, plasticity increases as one moves from A through D.

The search for a language module may be construed as a search for a type B module. Let us call such a type B language module an "elementary linguistic unit," or "ELU." It will also be remembered that in § 5.3, I provided a notation to describe the entities in view here. A true module (any of types A through C) is a certain sort of network of neurons, which I called an "M-network" (for convenience we may regard all of the types A through E as M-networks, even though the paradigm cases encompass only A through C). A "C-network" is the composite structure that brings the several modules implicated in a complex function into coalition. Language as a gross psychological capacity is mediated by a restricted class of C-networks (e.g., a speech comprehension network, a speech production network, etc.). This much is beyond dispute. The proponent of a language "module" needs to show in addition that at least one of these language C-networks' constituents is an ELU. Indeed, the traditional claim is more ambitious, with theorists maintaining that there is in effect a large M-network that handles core aspects of language—a super-sized ELU, as it were—such as Chomsky's Merge or Fodor's sentence parser (see later in this chapter) (Chomsky 1980a, pp. 39, 44, 1988, p. 159, 2002, pp. 84–86; Fodor 1983; Plaut 1995; Pinker & Jackendoff 2005, p. 207; Fitch et al. 2005, p. 182; Collins 2008, p. 155; Fedorenko & Thompson-Schill 2014). The argument of the present chapter is that there are unlikely to be *any* ELUs—that the only units we are likely to find among the constituents of our language C-networks are M-networks of the types C through E.

Now it may seem that this construal of the matter is austere, and that I have set a most demanding test for the modularity of language. Other ways of understanding linguistic modularization have occasionally been discussed. Broadly speaking, these fall into two categories, one of which might be called a "neurological" or "structural" understanding, the other a "psychological" one (by now a familiar distinction). The neurolinguists Evelina Fedorenko and Sharon Thompson-Schill (2014) explain them using network concepts. The structural notion is the more or less conventional one I have just described, which looks for an ELU. As they put it, "a network may be functionally specialized for mental process x if all of its nodes are functionally specialized for x, [but] perhaps the presence of at least one functionally specialized node is sufficient to qualify the whole network as functionally specialized" (2014, p. 121). In this view, even a single ELU would suffice as evidence of the specialization of language.

The psychological approach, on the other hand, would count as specialized any system whose pattern of interconnections between nodes is unique to the function the system performs:

> In this approach, the properties of the nodes are less important; they may be functionally specialized, domain general, or a mixture of the two. What matters is whether a unique combination of nodes and edges is recruited for the relevant mental process x. If so, such a network would be considered functionally specialized for x, even if all of the individual nodes are domain general . . . and even the same exact combination of nodes can contribute differently to different mental processes when the nodes are characterized by different patterns of connection. (Fedorenko & Thompson-Schill 2014, p. 121)

In this much more liberal view, language is specialized if the patterns of connections that characterize its C-networks are unique to those networks, notwithstanding that the same (indeed even the *very* same) nodes are recruited beyond the language domain, provided that the wiring patterns are distinctive in each case. Translated into psycholinguistic terms, a linguistic capacity (e.g., phoneme discrimination, lexical retrieval, etc.) would count as specialized and hence domain-specific if its representations were unique to the linguistic domain.[2] For example, if representations of speech sounds or lexical items are unique to language, in that they are consumed only while an agent is engaged in linguistic tasks, they would count as domain-specific. Intuitively, it will be easier to show that a capacity is domain-specific in this psychological sense than it will be in the neurological/structural sense: for it is unlikely that the linguistic representations involved in (say) phoneme discrimination, lexical retrieval, or syntactic parsing are consumed outside the specific contexts of linguistic communication. By the same logic, chess playing and golf will employ domain-specific representations. Of course, few would deny the importance of network configurations when explaining cognitive functions, or that there are occasions when our attention is properly captured by the dynamics of distinct (and in that sense, "specialized")

---

[2] See my earlier comments on domain specificity in § 4.2.3, and the discussion there more generally about "system" modules.

networks. But it would surely surprise no one that the brain enters into a different state whenever it switches between tasks, or even that such states are reasonably consistent across individuals. Systems specialized in this sense lack the stability and permanence underwriting the sort of specialization likely to be of interest to those in search of a language module. What has predominantly mattered to these researchers is just the extent to which mental processes like language rely on structurally dedicated mechanisms and specific computations.

John Collins, for instance (a philosopher and noted defender of generative linguistics), conjectures that "the peculiar specificity of language deficits suggests that the realization of language is found in dedicated circuitry, as opposed to more general levels of organization" (Collins 2008, p. 155). Chomsky himself has written that "It would be surprising indeed if we were to find that the principles governing [linguistic] phenomena are operative in other cognitive systems. . . . [T]here is good reason to suppose that the functioning of the language faculty is guided by special principles specific to this domain" (Chomsky 1980a, p. 44). Barely a decade later, he wrote that "[i]t would be astonishing if we were to discover that the constituent elements of the language faculty enter crucially in other domains" (Chomsky 1988, p. 159). Many commentators (e.g., Goldberg 2003; Pinker & Jackendoff 2005) frequently assume that Chomsky has relented in his stridency concerning this requirement, but in fact he has continued to hold out for the potential vindication of "earlier versions of generative grammar" in this regard (see, e.g., Fitch et al. 2005, p. 182, and the ambivalent remarks in Chomsky 2010, p. 53). For despite the abstractness of the Minimalist Program—which simplifies the idealization to language in the interests of evolutionary tractability—Chomsky has continued to write of a "language organ" that is "analogous to the heart or the visual system or the system of motor coordination and planning," commenting approvingly of the view that regards specialized learning mechanisms as "organs within the brain" that are "neural circuits whose structure enables them to perform one particular kind of computation" (Chomsky 2002, pp. 84–86). Thus linguistic specialization for Chomsky relates both to structure and to function, which is presumably why he continues to refer to "the radical (double) dissociations that have been found since [Eric] Lenneberg's pioneering work in the 1950s" (Chomsky 2018, p. 28). Pinker and Jackendoff (2005, p. 207) also defend something like this, pointing to neuroimaging and brain damage studies suggesting that "partly distinct sets of brain areas subserve speech and non-speech sounds," evidence that speech perception "dissociates in a number of ways from the perception of auditory events."

For this reason I have construed the issue of linguistic specialization along more traditional lines.[3] I turn next to the other aspect of the problem of defining a language module.

7.2.2 The domain of language clarified

In one sense, defining the language domain ought to be a simple affair, for is it not just the domain that encompasses activities such as speaking and signing, and (on a broader plane) reading and writing? The straightforward answer to this is yes, but the complete picture is somewhat more complicated by the deep and really rather mysterious relationship between thought and language. It is clear that language expresses a speaker's thoughts, and that whatever many other purposes a language may serve, it always comes down to the ability to convert sound (or some other signal) into meanings, and meanings into sound (Chomsky 1980b, p. 46; Sterelny 2006, p. 24; Jackendoff 2007, p. 2; Christiansen & Chater 2016, pp. 114–115). From this perspective, it is natural to view language as serving some sort of coding function, and the language faculty as a cognitive system that enables translation between "mentalese" and strings of symbols (Pinker 1994, p. 60). In such a view, there would seem to be at least two (potentially overlapping but functionally distinct) interacting systems of interest: a thought or "central" system on one hand, and a coding or translation system on the other.[4] One system generates and processes thoughts; the other encodes and decodes them. The second system takes its input from the first during production tasks, while the first takes its input from the second during comprehension tasks. This is admittedly crude and schematic; there are also many who would question

---

[3] Interestingly, Fedorenko and Thompson-Schill (2014, p. 122) discuss *and endorse* a third, dynamic (time- rather than task-centered) approach to specialization in which "the notion of functional specialization may be linked to the stability of the node/network; a network may be functionally specialized for some mental process if its nodes are stable community members and . . . domain general if its nodes frequently change allegiances." But this approach uses stability of activation over time as a guide to specialization in the *first* (neurological) sense, not the second (psychological) sense. In other words, their third approach is just that: an *approach* to identifying (neurologically/structurally) specialized brain regions within networks, rather than a definition of specialization *per se*. And the psychological sense is *not* specifically endorsed.

[4] Within the framework I have been pursuing here, these systems would be construed as two distinct (if possibly overlapping) C-networks.

the aptness of a conduit metaphor for language (Evans & Levinson 2009, pp. 435–436; Smit 2014). Nonetheless, I think the picture is reasonable. As Justin Leiber (2006, pp. 30–31) puts it, the "commonplace distinction that psychologists and linguists use [takes] speaking and hearing to be 'encoding' and 'decoding'—i.e., converting thoughts, or mental items, into the physical speech stream, and converting the physical speech stream into thoughts, or mental items." Certainly a more useful analogy in the present context would be hard to find, since disputants in the debate over linguistic modularity can be roughly grouped in accordance with how broadly they construe the language domain—as we shall see, there are those who would have it encompass (or even be reduced to) thought, and those who would restrict it to the coding function alone.

Chomsky's (1965, 1975, 1979, 1980a, 1995, 2002, 2005, 2010, 2016) many iterations of the language module have one thing in common in their portrayal of a central system that encompasses the very mechanisms of thought (Chomsky 2018; McGilvray 2014, p. 59; Collins 2004, p. 518). In a collaborative paper, Hauser, Chomsky and Fitch (2002) distinguished between the faculty of language in a narrow sense (FLN) from the faculty of language in a broad sense (FLB). FLN as a subset of the mechanisms underlying FLB is "the abstract linguistic computational system alone, independent of the other systems with which it interacts and interfaces" (Hauser et al. 2002, p. 1571). Their assumption is that "a key component of FLN is a computational system (narrow syntax) that generates internal representations and maps them into the sensory-motor interface by the phonological system, and into the conceptual-intentional interface by the (formal) semantic system" (Hauser et al. 2002, p. 1571). Furthermore, "a core property of FLN is recursion," which yields discrete infinity and is suggested to be the only uniquely human and uniquely linguistic cognitive possession (Hauser et al. 2002, p. 1571). The property of discrete infinity allows the generation of a limitless array of hierarchically structured expressions from a finite base of elements—the same property that (it is alleged) generates the system of natural numbers (Chomsky 2005, 2010). The technical term for this operation is "Merge," which in its simplest terms is just set formation (Berwick & Chomsky 2016, pp. 10, 98). Merge combines words ("Lexical Items") and sets of words, taking their semantic information ("features") to a semantic interface (SEM—the "conceptual-intentional system") and their sound information to a phonetic interface (PHON—the "sensory-motor system"). Merge is therefore a system that generates sentences ("expressions") in an inner symbolic code or language of thought (an "I-language") (Chomsky 2005, pp. 3, 4, 2010, pp. 55, 59; see also Chomsky 2018).

It is important to be clear about what conception of language lies behind this proposal. It is easy to be misled by talk of a phonetic interface, the mappings to that interface, and indeed the whole sensory-motor apparatus, which along with the semantic system is supposed to be a system for linking sound and meaning. This tends to imply that the production of an acoustic signal for the purpose of externalization and communication is what language is for. But this is actually only "the traditional assumption" (Chomsky 2010, p. 54). The "primary relation" of interest is supposed to be that between the core faculty of language (FLN) and SEM; i.e., the "systems of thought" (Chomsky 2010, pp. 54–55). Expressions that satisfy the interface conditions of SEM yield a "language of thought," and it is hypothesized that "the earliest stage of language," which supposedly arose prior to externalization, was "just that: a language of thought, available for use internally" (Chomsky 2010, p. 55). This inner code was the unique possession of a privileged individual, Prometheus, whose language provided him with "capacities for complex thought, planning, interpretation, and so on . . . [which] would then be transmitted to offspring, coming to predominate" (Chomsky 2010, p. 59). It is easy to forget that because externalization and communication came later, the language of Prometheus was not just a silent inner speech, as the residue of an internalized conventional public symbol system might be. Rather, it is hypothesized to be something like the reflexively complex but wordless stream of thought available to (presumably) any member of *Homo sapiens* not yet exposed to a public language.[5] For language is "virtually synonymous with symbolic thought" (Chomsky 2010, p. 59, quoting Ian Tattersall), and "fundamentally a system of thought" (Berwick & Chomsky 2016, p. 102). Perhaps the clearest indication that for Chomsky, language is the acme of central cognition, is recent remarks suggesting that language functions as a means of integrating information from various proprietary domains: "language is the *lingua franca* that binds together the different representations from geometric and nongeometric 'modules,' just as an 'inner mental tool' should. Being able to integrate a variety of perceptual cues and reason about them . . . would seem to have definite selective advantages" (Berwick & Chomsky, pp. 165–166). This makes Prometheus' language a "language of thought" in pretty much the classical sense (Fodor 1975). Thus, when

---

[5] By "wordless" I mean without the words of a public language.

Chomsky implores us to consider how difficult it is *not* to talk to ourselves, both during sleep and our almost every waking hour (Berwick & Chomsky 2016, p. 64), to press the point that language is really an instrument of thought, it is important not to assume (no matter how reasonably) that he is extolling the virtues of a public language. The powerful scaffolding a public language provides in the form of an echo for our ideas and ruminations—the chance to objectify and insinuate our thoughts into a manipulatable format external to ourselves, surely what makes language able to serve as a "tool for thought" *par excellence*—cannot be denied, of course, and Chomsky certainly does not (e.g., Berwick & Chomsky, p. 102). But his primary aim here is not to make the case for externalization so much as to point up the intimate and virtually indissoluble relation between a Promethean private language and internal thought. For language here *ultimately* means something other than what most people, and I suspect what most language researchers, think about when they think about language (see later, this chapter). Most researchers would understand the coding function to be a distinct system for the translation of thought into the sentences of a public language, even if this system can be decomposed into elements that are shared with other systems (including systems of thought). Now just what all this implies for an ELU we shall come to presently, but first let me contrast Chomsky's view with Jerry Fodor's, who seems to have a more conventional—Chomsky would say "traditional"—understanding of what I have called the coding function.

Fodor has consistently maintained that only peripheral input systems are likely to be modular. In this view, modules are associated with specific channels of sensory transduction—there may be modules for vision, olfaction, and even aspects of syntactic processing, but probably not for complex thought, memory, and judgment. I have two points to make about this, the first somewhat ancillary to the second. In light of what I have discussed in previous chapters, *this* way of construing the difference between central and peripheral systems seems definitely mistaken. The material I presented in Chapters 2 through 5 demonstrates that elements of even our most evolutionarily ancient transduction systems participate in various cross-domain functional composites (C-networks), including those underlying central processes. Transduction dynamics, which are usually characterized by a certain degree of speed, autonomy, or reflexivity, may even be activated in many cases by the same domain-general nodes (M-networks/modules) that yield central system dynamics. This might in fact explain the frequent penetrability of perception. Thus it is no longer really plausible to cash out the difference between central and peripheral system dynamics in terms of modules, for just the same sorts of entities seem to underlie both types. Of course, Fodor does not in specific terms exclude the possibility that cognition might be underwritten by anatomically or functionally exiguous units throughout—the basic assumption in cognitive neuroscience. It is just that he has construed the term "module" to mean something quite specific: a device for the processing of transduced information. This construal simply does not contemplate the autonomous, domain-general columns that handle low-level subfunctions right across the neocortex, long understood to be the seat of complex thought and executive function. But Fodor does not own the term, and the modular hypothesis—under that very name and always referring to the functionally specialized units of the mind/brain—goes back at least to the 1950s, appearing in works by Vernon Mountcastle (1957, 1978), David Marr (1976), and Noam Chomsky (1980a) well before the appearance of Fodor's (1983) monograph.[6] As Collins (2004, p. 506) summarizes the Fodorian attitude to the central systems: "for Fodor, whether there are 'central' modules is at best moot; the thesis that *it's all modules* he considers to be virtually *a priori* false."

The point about Fodorian modularity I want to emphasize, however, is not that I think it draws a distinction that is somewhat arbitrary at the level of modularity (it may be more aptly drawn at some other level of inquiry; e.g., an evolutionary one); it is that his understanding of modularity leads directly to a certain kind of language module, one very different from Chomsky's (Collins 2004). Since modules for him are peripheral input devices, it follows that any language module must be peripheral, and thus *not* the sort of system that generates expressions in an inner symbolic code, as Chomsky's does. Fodor's language module is a "sentence encoding-decoding system"—a parser, with an encapsulated representation of grammar (Fodor et al. 1974, p. 370).[7] Language is for him "a psychological mechanism that can be plausibly thought of as functioning to provide information about the distal environment in a format appropriate for central processing" (Fodor 1983, p. 44). In this account, language is not a central process, not pure symbolic thought, as it is for Chomsky; rather it is a "psychological mechanism" that provides

---

[6] I do accept, of course, that Fodor performed a tremendous service in shaping the discussion of modularity in cognitive psychology.

[7] "A speech episode involves the encoding and decoding of an internal representation of a sentence.... [I]t is clear that a very complex coding system mediates between the internal representation and the speech event" (Fodor et al. 1974, p. 21).

grist for the central system mill (i.e., for the inner "language of thought"). The cleavage between Chomsky and Fodor, then, relates to the difference between "knowledge" and "use" of language, or "competence" and "performance" (Chomsky 2018). Chomsky's module is an internal generative device that accounts for our *knowledge* of language (competence). Fodor's is a peripheral input device that accounts for our *use* of language (performance).

All this can make for confusion in debates about the modularity of language. It is not hard to see how interlocutors might talk past one another. Does a mechanism recruited exclusively for thought, or perhaps for thought and a more peripheral coding operation—but nowhere else across cognition—count as an ELU? Or must the mechanism be exclusive to the coding operation alone before it can be considered an ELU? It depends on whether you view systems of thought as forming part of the domain of language. Evidently some do and others do not. Take metarepresentation as a case in point: the capacity for nested thinking that allows us to embed thoughts within thoughts, in principle indefinitely, witnessed in a child's being able to draw a picture of themselves drawing a picture (Suddendorf 2013; Zerilli 2014). If it could be shown that metarepresentation is an exclusive property of thought, or an exclusive property of thought and the coding function taken together, metarepresentation would count as an ELU in a Chomskian interpretation of language (defined in terms of thought). For someone with a more traditional understanding, in contrast, metarepresentation would not count as an ELU, for although it might appear in the coding function, it is exploited outside the language domain (defined in terms of processes that operate distinctly from thought), in this case within the systems of thought.

Morten Christiansen and Nick Chater are two psycholinguists who appear to have the more traditional understanding of the language domain in mind. Among the various factors they cite to explain why natural languages appear to be so well suited to the human brain, and hence easy to learn and process, they include "constraints from thought" (Christiansen & Chater 2016, p. 51). This form of explanation makes most sense from the point of view that language and thought are not synonymous (otherwise the explanation would be uninformative). It is just as well, then, that Christiansen and Chater do indeed regard "constraints from thought" as "non-linguistic constraints" (2016, p. 50). To give a vivid sense of the confusion that these differences of view have engendered, compare Christiansen and Chater's (2016) book with Berwick and Chomsky's (2016) book. Berwick and Chomsky maintain that "Universal Grammar" is language-specific, whereas Christiansen and Chater deny that the core operations in language processing abilities are language-specific, seeing them as merely applications of general-purpose, non-hierarchical, sequence learning abilities. However, as Richard Moore (2017, p. 611) pointed out in his illuminating review, "the nature of [the] disagreement here must be stated carefully because of the different ways in which BC and CC use the word 'language.'" He goes on:

> BC think that language, in the form of the conjunction of Merge and the conceptual interface, is an element of thought that underwent natural selection for improvements in planning. While for them language is independent of communication, for CC language is just the set of natural languages—and their use of the word reflects this. Given their view, BC would not expect that areas of the brain involved in natural language use would be used only for natural language; they will be used for general purpose thinking too. This makes their thesis less easy to distinguish from CC's. . . . If language is understood in terms of natural language, then neither BC nor CC hold that syntax is language-specific. (Moore 2017, pp. 611–612)

If the interlocutors themselves paid more attention to these distinctions, the precise nature of their disagreements could be better understood.

While I shall adopt the more traditional construal of the language domain (*à la* Christiansen and Chater), in § 7.3 I will survey evidence of the extensive reuse of language circuits across domains having nothing much to do with either language *or* thought. In other words, the material I present herein should be problematic for *anyone* defending the existence of an ELU, regardless of how eccentrically they wish to construe the language domain.

7.2.3 Examples of elementary linguistic units

Before leaving this section, I should provide some further guidance on the most likely candidates for the role of an ELU. Now that we have clarified both in what respects an ELU would be specialized and in what sense it could be linguistic, we can turn to some concrete proposals.

Much of the impetus for the claim that the mind/brain contains ELUs came from early work in generative linguistics, which formalized a large stock of highly intricate and apparently system-specific rules for the derivation of grammatical strings ("surface structures") from the more abstract "kernel" sentences ("deep structures") underlying them (Chomsky 1956, 1957). These unspoken deep structures were hypothesized to be "present to the mind" whenever a speaker produces the surface forms of her language (Chomsky 2006, p. 16). This inspired the belief that the mind/brain incorporates specialized systems that function more or less exclusively for the generation of surface structures. While the field of generative linguistics today would hardly be recognizable to an undergraduate familiar with work from (say) the mid–late 1960s, the influence of that early work has not dissipated entirely—and it is, for all that times have changed, still plausible to suppose that at least some linguistic operations are domain-specific. Let me illustrate with a simple example drawn from the generative tradition.

The assignment of phonetic interpretations to surface structures might hint at cognitive resources that, by virtue of how detailed and context-specific they seem, could reasonably be supposed to serve no other function. Assume that a speaker has encountered the following phonetic realizations:

expedite → expeditious
contrite → contrition
ignite → ignition

Assume further that the speaker has not yet encountered the word "righteous," so has not yet been in a position to establish the derivation

right → righteous

The speaker on hearing "righteous" (properly so as "rahy-chuh-s") for the first time knows that the underlying form cannot be the same as for expeditious, contrition, and so on (unless the case is just an exception), though had the speaker heard "rish-uh-s" they would not have hesitated in concluding that "rite" would be the underlying form (analogously to expedite/expeditious, etc.). The speaker understands that the underlying form of "righteous" must instead be "right" (or, more technically, a form containing "i" followed by the velar continuant "gh"), for only some such form could make sense of what was heard given the following rule (which the speaker must be taken to know):

"t" followed by a high front vowel ["-eou," "-iou," "-ion," "-ian," etc.] is realized as "ch" [as in *ch*ew, *ch*oke, *ch*allenge, etc.] after a continuant [e.g.,

"–ahy," as in f*igh*t, b*igh*t, s*igh*t, etc.—as opposed to "i" as in f*i*t, b*i*t, s*i*t, etc.], and as "sh" [as in *sh*oe, *sh*ow, *sh*am, etc.] elsewhere.

Detailed phonological rules of this kind—in fact much more intricate ones than this—have frequently been thought to reflect principles not obviously assimilable to other cognitive domains, pertaining exclusively to the coding function. This accompanies the thought that such rules are so exotic as far as the agent's overall envelope of capacities go that handling them must require a very special suite of neural and computational resources.

Pinker and Jackendoff (2005) suggest other rules. They observe that many grammatical principles have no real application outside language, principles such as linear word order (*John loves Mary*/*Mary loves John*), agreement (*the boy runs* vs *the boy run*), case (*John saw him* vs *John saw he*), tense, aspect, derivational morphology (*run*/*runner*), and inflectional morphology (*the girls are*/*the girl is*). Moreover, they contend that linguistic recursivity is not reducible to analogues in mathematics. They also nominate speech perception as possibly uniquely adapted for the perception of human speech sounds (and not other types of sounds). Brattico and Liikkanen (2009, p. 261), in passing, suggest that the lexicon, as "a list of feature bundles," is domain-specific. Their argument is in fact that the only truly domain-specific aspects of language will turn out to be nongenerative—generative mechanisms (recursion/Merge) will be domain-general. Once again, though, it is not always clear what is meant by "domain-specific." While Pinker and Jackendoff seem to have the more robust sense of dissociability in view—that is, at least in part a structural notion—one could interpret "domain-specific lexicon" to imply merely that lexical *representations* are domain-specific, a considerably weaker notion. To be clear (and at the risk of repetition), it is only the former (structural) notion that interests me here.

Actually, the question of what it takes to be domain-specific, or "specialized for X," can be a little more complicated. For instance, associative learning is the paradigm domain-general cognitive capacity (in both the structural and psychological senses). But a particular learned association, say between fire and warmth, could be considered domain-specific in yet another (somewhat misleading) sense: the specific associative mechanism linking fire and warmth may be discretely localized in the brain and active only in response to those specific stimuli. Similarly, we might have a general capacity to run recursive algorithms, but a parallel implementation of that procedure, say a numerical one, would be "domain-specific." It is therefore important to distinguish between a general capacity, and a specific, repeated and (potentially) parallel use of that capacity. I will return to this important distinction in § 7.5 when I discuss neural redundancy.

7.3 *Is* There a Language Module?

As we saw in Chapter 4, certain areas of the brain have long been regarded as quintessentially language areas. For many researchers this assumption and the conviction that there is far more nature than nurture involved in language acquisition have sat cheek by jowl. In the last two decades, however, the standard view of how language is organized and processed in the brain, as well as how it is acquired, has changed dramatically. This is so for at least two reasons (Kuhl & Damasio 2013). First, neuroimaging evidence in the form of electroencephalography, magnetoencephalography, positron emission tomography, and (increasingly) functional magnetic resonance imaging has furnished a wealth of information about how and where language is processed in real time in the brains of patients carrying out linguistic tasks. The picture that emerges here is very unlike the one bequeathed by Paul Broca and Carl Wernicke. Second, psycholinguistic evidence is much richer and subtler than what was available in previous decades. It reveals that infants begin learning language from the moment they come into contact with the sound inventories of their native tongue, indeed, even *in utero*. It appears that the early sensitivity of a fetus to features of intonation may later help the infant learn its mother tongue (Mampe et al. 2009). For instance, the French "papa" has a delayed stress, and a rising intonation, while the German has an early stress, and a falling intonation. When an infant begins to form its first sounds, it can build on melodic patterns that are thus already familiar, and so does not have to start from scratch when learning phonological and morphological regularities (the investigators suspect the evolutionary roots of this behavior to be older than the emergence of spoken language). I shall say a little more on the acquisition issue in my next section. Here I shall focus on organization, and review evidence of the extensive reuse of what were traditionally regarded typical language circuits.

Plausibly, the more distributed a system in the brain, the more likely it is that it will *not* be a specialized system (Anderson 2010; see my Chapter 3). It is now known that language is one of the most distributed systems in the brain, and that "the operation of language to its full extent requires a much more extended network than what [classical models have] assumed" (Hagoort & Indefrey 2014, p. 359; Anderson 2010, p. 247). As Hagoort and Indefrey summarized the emerging consensus:

> The basic principle of brain organization for higher cognitive functions proposes that these functions are based on the interaction between numerous neuronal circuits and brain regions that support various contributing functional components. These circuits are not necessarily specialized for language but nevertheless need to be recruited for the sake of successful language processing. (2014, p. 359)

The evidence motivating this principle in turn corroborates the prediction that more recently evolved functions should be more distributed than older ones, since it should overall prove easier to exploit existing circuits than to have to evolve custom-made ones, with there being "little reason to suppose that the useful elements will happen to reside in neighboring brain regions. . . . [A] more localist account of the evolution of the brain would . . . expect the continual development of new, largely dedicated neural circuits" for new functions (Anderson 2010, p. 246). Anderson's review of some 1500 subtraction-based fMRI experiments suggests that language could well be the paradigm of distributed processing, supported by more distributed activations than visual perception and attention are (Anderson 2007a) and indeed than any other domain that was tested, including reasoning, memory, emotion, mental imagery, and action (Anderson 2008).

Broca's area holds a special place in the tradition of modular theorizing about language. While it cannot be doubted that the area plays a crucial role in language processing, it is also implicated in various action- and imagery-related tasks such as those involving the preparation of movement (Thoenissen et al. 2002), the sequencing of actions (Nishitani et al. 2005), the recognition of actions (Decety et al. 1997; Nishitani et al. 2005), imagery of motion (Binkofski et al. 2000), and the imitation of actions (Nishitani et al. 2005). It is also known to be involved in certain memory tasks (Kaan & Stowe 2002) as well as in music perception (Maess et al. 2001). Kaan and Swaab (2002) set out to identify whether syntactic processing is localized in the brain, and found that while Broca's area is recruited during syntactic processing tasks, it joins a larger brain network that includes the anterior, middle, and superior areas of the temporal lobes, none of which in turn appears to be syntax-specific.

In the auditory domain, phoneme discrimination has long impressed perceptual psychologists. It involves "categorical perception"; that is, "the segmenting of a signal that varies continuously along a number of physical dimensions . . . into discrete categories, so that signals within the category are counted as the same, even though acoustically, they may differ from one another more than do two signals in different categories" (Cowie 2008, at § 3.3.4). Fiona Cowie, no fan of linguistic nativism, accepts that there is a "quite substantial . . . inborn contribution to phonological learning." But, as she goes on to discuss:

> . . . is this inborn contribution to phonological learning *language spe-cific*[?]. . . . [T]o this question, the answer appears to be "No." First, the "chunking" of continuously varying stimuli into discrete categories is a feature not just of speech perception, but of human perception generally. For instance, it has been demonstrated in the perception of non-linguistic sounds, like musical pitch, key and melody, and meaningless chirps and bleats. . . . It has also been demonstrated in the processing of visual stimuli like faces. . . . Secondly, it is known that other animals too perceive categorically. For instance, crickets segment conspecific songs in terms of frequency . . . swamp sparrows "chunk" notes of differing durations. . . . [O]ther species respond categorically to human speech! Chinchillas . . . and cotton-top tamarins . . . make similar phonological distinctions to those made by human infants. (Cowie 2008, at § 3.3.4)

A recent experiment found that early exposure to multiple languages heightens acoustic sensitivity generally (Liu & Kager 2016). In particular, bilingual children appear more sensitive to subtle variations in musical pitch than their monolingual counterparts.

There is something especially piquant in discovering that classic sensory and motor areas play a key role in higher thought. In Chapter 2, I reviewed evidence of the role of vision in semantics. Damasio and Martin demonstrated over two decades ago that visual areas are active during noun-processing tasks (e.g., naming colors, animals, etc.) (Damasio & Tranel 1993; Damasio et al. 1996; Martin et al. 1995, 1996, 2000). We saw that word-generation in sighted subjects depends at least in part on the bilateral occipital cortices, regions that have always been thought to be the most specialized in the brain (Pascual-Leone et al. 2005, p. 394). Beyond the association with phylogenetically older sensory and perceptual functions, language also seems to have been originally bound up with the motor system, for motor circuits still appear to be crucial to language perception and comprehension on many levels of processing (as indeed the functional profile of Broca's area would tend to suggest). Pulvermüller and Fadiga (2010) report that at the level of speech perception and processing, changes in the motor and premotor cortex lead to deficits in phoneme discrimination (2010, pp. 353–355). There is also evidence that the acoustic properties of phonemes have been shaped to some extent by postural aspects of the motor system (Graziano et al. 2002; MacNeilage 1998). At the level of semantic comprehension, magnetic stimulation of the motor system influences the recognition of semantic word categories (Pulvermüller & Fadiga 2010, pp. 355–357). Pulvermüller (2005) earlier reported evidence that hearing the words "lick," "pick" and "kick," in that order, activates successively more of the primary motor cortex, suggesting both that the motor regions involved are inherent to the comprehension task and that comprehension may involve some kind of simulation. Glenberg et al. (2008) report similar findings, in particular how the use-driven plasticity of motor circuits affects abstract and concrete language processing. Incidentally, it has been demonstrated that reading comprehension improves when children are allowed to manipulate physical objects (Glenberg et al. 2007). Finally, syntactic processing seems to depend in important ways upon the perisylvian cortex, which is involved in the processing of hierarchically structured action sequences (e.g., lifting a cup, turning it this way, etc., as guided by the overall aim of quenching thirst) (Pulvermüller & Fadiga 2010, pp. 357–358). And it is known that both word- and object-combining have overlapping neural implementations (Greenfield 1991). (I review more evidence of the motor–syntax connection in my discussion of sequence learning later in this chapter.) Taken together, these results suggest that the motor system enters nontrivially into the perception and comprehension of language at various levels of processing, including phonological, semantic, and syntactic levels (Knott 2012).

This brings us back to Broca's area. I have already reviewed evidence attesting to its functional complexity and its importance in action sequencing. A natural response of those committed to the specificity of language circuits would be to concede all of this reuse, and say simply that what we are witnessing is the reuse of *linguistic* circuits for other, nonlinguistic functions. A subtle variant of this idea lies behind the contention that Merge may be the source of productivity and generativity in nonlinguistic domains. As Brattico and Liikkanen pose the issue:

To how many cognitive domains can this combinatorial operation be applied? In principle, there seems to be no limit, provided that the appropriate interface mechanisms are in place. This architecture of language makes it easy to imagine a recursive symbol processor which can create productive behavior in several cognitive domains depending on which type of symbols it applies to and which type of interfaces it is required to handle. (2009, p. 262)

Following Chomsky, they opine that it might have been the application of Merge to concepts that yielded the "explosive growth of the capacities of thought . . . leading to the liberty of the imagination to transpose and change its ideas," which, as suggested by Hume, could generate such imaginary objects as "winged horses, fiery dragons, and monstrous giants." When Merge is emptied of all content, the result is the system of natural numbers.[8] And so on. The research just mentioned, highlighting the indispensable contribution of primitive sensory-motor areas for syntactic and semantic processing, suggests that the argument is skewed, for it tends to imply that Merge, recursion, metarepresentation, or whatever generative engine happens to be invoked to account for linguistic productivity—with Broca's area providing its most likely neurological basis (see, e.g., Brattico & Liikkanen 2009, p. 273)—is some sort of ELU; i.e., an integrated, dedicated, self-contained computational mechanism, perhaps dissociable from core motor operations (see, e.g., Berwick & Chomsky 2016, pp. 75–77). If far more evolutionarily primitive mechanisms are behind crucial aspects of linguistic processing at the highest levels, this seems very suppositious. It is more plausible (i.e., parsimonious) to assume that linguistic productivity was assembled from prior sensory-motor materials, with Broca's area providing a rich source of sequence-processing power (see further in this chapter). That is to say, the role of Broca's area in language is evidence that it *already* performed just the kind of sensory-motor functions that made it ideal for integration within a larger language network (Müller & Basho 2004).

This conjecture is rendered more plausible when one reflects further on the deep connections between syntactic structure and motor sequences.[9] Even in lower organisms, motion is never haphazard and shambolic; it is always coordinated, structured, and systematic relative to the organism's

---

[8] "It is not hard to show that, if the lexicon is reduced to a single element, then Merge will yield a form of arithmetic" (Chomsky 2010, p. 53).

[9] For a sophisticated and fully developed computational account, see Knott (2012).

aims and the needs of survival. Coordination is intrinsic to motor function, a basic prerequisite of meaningful action. Basic body acts form "action chains" of "meaningful goal-directed action sequence[s]," as exemplified in the drinking-from-a-cup action sequence mentioned earlier (Pulvermüller and Fadiga 2010, p. 357). A center-embedded sentence (The man {whom the dog chased away} ran away) parallels the nested structure of a typical jazz piece (theme {solo} modified theme) and the action chain formed when entering a dark room at night (open the door {switch on the light} close the door); in each of these cases, "a superordinate sequence surrounds a nested action or sequence" (Pulvermüller and Fadiga 2010, p. 357). Indeed, the patterns of coordination and subordination within many complex/cumulative sentences are often deliberately designed to evoke the actions they describe, a device familiar to writers and on display in the best literature (Landon 2013). It should not come as a surprise, then, that syntax recruits the same areas of the brain that are essential for the planning and coordination of movement. Christiansen and Chater (2016) go a little further, placing sequence learning at center-stage of their account of linguistic productivity. They think complex sequence learning amply explains our ability to process recursive structures, and (consistent with my theme) that recursivity "relies on evolutionarily older abilities for dealing with temporally presented sequences of input" (2016, p. 204). There is a wealth of comparative and genetic evidence—quite apart from the neural evidence I have dwelt on up to this point—that can also be marshalled in support of the idea that language makes heavy demands on our complex sequence-learning abilities. What is currently known of the *FOXP2* gene is consistent with a human adaptation for sequential processing (Fisher & Scharff 2009). It is well known that mutations of the gene produce severe speech and orofacial impairments (Lai et al. 2001; MacDermot et al. 2005). Moreover, when the homologous gene was inserted into mice, the mice displayed superior learning abilities for action sequences (Schreiweis et al. 2014). Specific language impairment (SLI), for its part, seems to be the result of a clear sequence-processing deficit (Hsu et al. 2014). Further neural evidence of a shared basis for language and general sequence learning is also available (see the review in Christiansen & Chater 2016, pp. 206–207). For example, syntactic and sequencing abilities do not appear to dissociate: when one gets knocked out, chances are the other does, too.

Notice, by the way, that (without prejudging the issue) this account is compatible with the idea that aspects of arithmetic, conceptual thought, musical syntax, and so on, could be exaptations of prior sequence-learning capabilities, whether via language or some other (perhaps more direct) phylogenetic route. Certainly recursive and metarepresentational capacities seem to crop up elsewhere in cognition, well outside the domains of language and thought, such as mental time travel, theory of mind/sociality, culture, and morality (Suddendorf 2013).

Thus far I have been largely concerned with the neuroimaging and biobehavioral evidence against linguistic modularity. For the remainder of this section, I shall very briefly mention a few arguments based on other considerations; namely, those arising from evolutionary theory and computational modeling. In the upcoming section, I shall address the matter of innateness. The final section introduces my Redundancy Model to account for the rare but still important evidence of cognitive dissociations, as well as other phenomena not easily explicable without some such account.

It is widely accepted that, of all human phenotypes, language is one of relatively recent origin, certainly far more recently evolved than basic sensory-motor, memory, and conceptual systems. Even if one adopts the view that language and the physiological mechanisms required to support complex vocalizations evolved together (i.e., that language and speech co-evolved), by any account, language is a phylogenetically recent phenomenon—de Boer (2016) thinks it is as old as the adaptations for complex vocalizations and places its emergence at around 400,000 years ago. This fact at once suggests that specific cognitive adaptations for language are unlikely, essentially for the reasons already given: it is generally easier for evolution to reuse and exapt existing resources than to have to evolve them from scratch (Anderson 2010). But other reasons support this conclusion as well. For adaptations to arise, evolution requires a stable environment (Sterelny 2006; Christiansen & Chater 2016). An adaptation for language would require a *linguistically* stable environment, but language and cultural environments generally are anything but stable, with both words and structural features of languages subject to swift changes, and cultures subject to significant shifts of convention, often even intragenerationally (Dunn et al. 2011; Greenhill et al. 2010; Sterelny 2012). In fact, when it comes to cultural environments, *plasticity* is typically favored over robustness—changes that allow the organism to cope with unpredictable variations in the local environment are favored over specific adaptations narrowly tailored to that environment, unless of course the culture *does* provide a stable target over which selection can operate (see § 7.4).

Changing tack somewhat, advances in computational neuroscience have uncovered a core set of standard, "canonical" neural computations. These computations are "combined and repeated across brain regions and modalities to apply similar operations to different problems" (Carandini 2015, p. 179). One example of a canonical computation, particularly in sensory systems, is "filtering." This is a basic connectionist operation in which neurons perform a weighted sum on sensory inputs. The weights are called "receptive fields," and the process is performed across the visual, auditory, somatosensory, and possibly motor systems—systems most of which we have seen are important and even crucial to language processing. Another canonical computation is "divisive normalization." This involves dividing neuronal responses by a common factor; namely, the summed activity of a specific collection of neurons. The process is considered important to operations as varied as "the representation of odours, the deployment of visual attention, the encoding of value, and the integration of multisensory information" (Carandini 2015, p. 180). Other examples would include predictive coding, which has certainly received its fair share of attention in recent years (Clark 2013), as well as "exponentiation, recurrent amplification, associative learning rules, cognitive maps, coincidence detection, top-down gain changes, population vectors, and constrained trajectories in dynamical systems" (Carandini 2015, p. 180). What all this shows is that, at levels of explanation not too far down—we are still at the "algorithmic" level here, not quite yet at the circuit or cell level—there are fundamental computations intrinsic to the functioning of the brain that cut across various modalities, very probably including language. Cognitive operations thus look set to share many of their underlying computations with other domains, even with domains whose physical resources they do not actually share.

While we are on the topic, it might be good to mention Spaun again (the brain simulation we met in Chapter 3). Spaun makes a different point, one I have been at pains to make in this section, this chapter, and indeed throughout the whole book. Spaun has been successful in showing that a computer can employ fully domain-general learning principles, for Spaun *reuses* the same circuits to accomplish very different functions (cf. Pinker 1994). As I explained in Chapter 3, most machines are good at doing just one thing (playing chess, solving equations, etc.). Spaun is unique both in the variety of the tasks it can perform and in its ability to learn new tasks using the same set of circuits. It is the first major step in answering an important challenge leveled by evolutionary psychologists and other proponents of traditional forms of modularity who for many years said that such a machine could not be designed (virtually on a priori grounds!). Well, Spaun is a machine that functions entirely by domain-general principles. (*Quod erat demonstrandum.*)

7.4 Is Language Innate?

Let me begin with a couple of straightforward observations. Infants begin their lives with a remarkable ability to detect and respond to subtle acoustic distinctions that vary considerably across the world's languages. Within a short time—indeed, before 10 months of age (Kuhl & Damasio 2013)—and pursuant to a powerful and in some respects still mysterious learning process, they come to recognize statistical properties in the acoustic stream, form phonetic categories, distill words and possibly inflectional items, and assimilate the basic phrase structure of their mother tongue. By one year of age, they appear able to comprehend simple imperatives like "Show me your nose" (Glickstein 2014). And even though the linguistic environment is not so impoverished as was once believed (Clark 2009, p. 368; Pullum & Scholz 2002; Scholz & Pullum 2002), it is still striking that most, if not all, of this gets underway without explicit instruction or drilling. Overall, adopting the terminology and concepts introduced in Chapter 6, let us admit that language acquisition involves a certain degree of *developmental robustness*—not quite like that of the visual system or the growth of wings on birds (or the growth of limbs, or the onset of puberty, or any of the other rhetorical claims made in the past), but something to reckon with, nonetheless. The appeal of a concept like robustness is that it admits of degrees, so that to confess that a system is characterized by robustness does not commit one to implausible claims. Actually, developmental robustness is somewhat reminiscent of the notion of being acquired under a "poverty of stimulus," because to be so acquired just *is* to develop independently of the presence of some specific environmental stimulus or stimuli, and hence denotes a sort of invariance with respect to experience (Griffiths & Machery 2008, pp. 406–407). Drawing this link is acceptable as long as the locution is employed with care, and with the understanding that acquisition under poverty of stimulus is a *relative* phenomenon, not an absolute one (see Chapter 6).

The question now is whether this developmental profile reopens the debate over the existence of an ELU. Does the fact that language seems to be acquired so early in life, with fair uniformity over substantial variations of intelligence and experience, without specific training, and so on, call for the postulation of a domain-specific language module? The move is reasonable, but unnecessary, for several reasons. It is worth remembering that however robust language acquisition might be, even in the most ideal conditions it can take a long time to complete (up to ten years or more). There is anyway a more natural and parsimonious explanation for why language acquisition proceeds at the ontogenetic pace it does, and why it often seems that children attain mastery of their native language almost effortlessly. The explanation lies in the mutual accommodation (or *fit*) between the processing dispositions of the brain regions used in language and language itself. There is evidence both that language was culturally shaped (as a "cultural tool") to be learnable and easy to process through cultural evolution (Everett 2012; Christiansen & Chater 2016; Laland 2016) and that selective pressures in the course of biological evolution may have equipped the brain with the sorts of processing dispositions and biases that made language easier to learn and process (Dor & Jablonka 2010; Sterelny 2006; Christiansen & Chater 2016; see also Laland et al. 2015). Since cultural evolution is much the most important side of this story, I shall have a little more to say about that than about biological evolution. But before I go any further, let me frame the main point of this section in terms of Stanislas Dehaene's (2005) "neuronal recycling" hypothesis, which we met briefly in Chapter 3.

Recall that towards the end of Chapter 6, I observed that while there is a relative sense in which modules and other functionally significant brain regions can be considered innate, the same cannot be said for the higher-level cognitive functions composed of them. Cast in terms of reuse, low-level cognitive *workings* may be innate, but it does not follow from this that higher-level cognitive *uses* are innate. Most complex cognitive functions are learned throughout the course of a person's life—whether it be riding a bicycle, tying one's shoes, or reading, these skills do not spontaneously unfurl as a result of intrinsically determined developmental processes, so it makes sense to withhold the designation "innate" or "robust" from the C-networks that implement them. Why, then, is language acquisition different from reading, performing long division, or learning physics? What is it about conversation that entitles us to regard *it* (and its C-network) as in some sense sharing in or inheriting the robustness of its components (workings/M-networks)? This is where Dehaene's notion of a "neuronal niche" is useful. Cultural acquisitions must make their home among a particular ensemble of cortical regions (a C-network), and this process is akin to the process of organisms' creating their own ecological niches among the habitats in which they find themselves. Just as organisms must make the best use of the resources at their disposal, so cognitive organisms (i.e., cultural acquisitions) are constrained by the processing dispositions of the brain regions required for the tasks at hand. We have already seen that brain regions *do* have robust processing capabilities and clear input preferences. Dehaene's idea is that the more the acquired practice matches the processing dispositions of the brain regions recruited for the task, the easier and less disruptive the learning process, because the neural composite does not require a radical departure from existing cortical biases. On the other hand, the greater the distance between the acquired practice and the processing dispositions of the brain regions it will draw upon, the more difficult and protracted the learning process will be, potentially disrupting the regions' established operations and whatever functional composites they already subserve.

It is not hard to see how this account would dovetail nicely with a cultural evolutionary account revealing the ways in which language has been shaped over many hundreds of generations to be learnable and easy to process. If human languages have in fact been so worked upon as to make them easy to learn and use, the neuronal niche that languages must nuzzle into already ideally conforms to the sorts of processing demands that languages impose on language users. It is just as well, then, that there is just such a cultural story to tell! Brighton et al. (2005) call it "cultural selection for learnability." If the rudiments of syntax, phonology, morphology, and so on are to survive from one generation to the next, they must earn their keep. If they are too cumbersome or exotic to be readily learned, taken up, and transmitted to the next generation, they will be discarded for simpler and more streamlined or efficient devices. There is mathematical modeling to suggest that compositionality could have evolved in this fashion, for instance (Smith & Kirby 2008; Kirby et al. 2007).

It is hard to deny that human languages are cultural products (Everett 2012). And if so, it makes perfect sense that they will reflect the cognitive and neural dispositions of the agents that created them in their own image. As Christiansen and Chater (2016, pp. 43–44) explain:

In other cultural domains, this is a familiar observation. Musical patterns appear to be rooted, in part at least, in the machinery of the human auditory and motor systems . . . art is partially shaped by the properties of human

> visual perception . . . tools, such as scissors or spades, are built around the constraints of the human body; aspects of religious beliefs may connect, among other things, with the human propensity for folk-psychological explanation.

They identify and elaborate upon four groups of nonlinguistic constraints that they conjecture would have guided the cultural evolution of language. (Much of this can be read as a natural extension of the ideas in § 7.3 concerning the reuse of language circuits.) They divide the constraints here between those arising from thought, perceptuo-motor factors, memory, and pragmatics. For example, on the assumption that thought is "prior to, and independent of, linguistic communication," key properties of language such as compositionality, predicate–argument structure, quantification, aspect, and modality can be "proposed to arise from the structure of the thoughts language is required to express" (2016, p. 51). Cognitive linguists have made the dependence of language on thought a critical feature of their perspective, arguing that our basic conceptual repertoire, including space and time, can be seen to have left their mark on the structure and categories of the world's languages (Croft & Cruise 2004; Evans & Green 2006). Perceptuo-motor constraints have also left their mark, most obviously in "the seriality of vocal output," which "forces a sequential construction of messages" (2016, p. 52). Christiansen and Chater speculate that

> The noisiness and variability . . . of vocal . . . signals may, moreover, force a "digital" communication system with a small number of basic messages: e.g., one that uses discrete units (phonetic features, phonemes, or syllables). The basic phonetic inventory is transparently related to deployment of the vocal apparatus, and it is also possible that it is tuned, to some degree, to respect "natural" perceptual boundaries. (2016, p. 52)

The extent of the connections here can be taken quite far. MacNeilage (1998), for example, has offered the intriguing hypothesis that syllabic structure might have been partly determined by the jaw movements involved in mastication! While not immediately obvious, on reflection it seems likely that many complex aspects of phonology and morphology will be traced to similarly prosaic origins. Memory constraints are hardly less significant; seen, for instance, in the tendency to resolve linguistic dependencies (e.g., between arguments and their verbs) as early as possible, "a tendency that might not be syntax-specific, but instead an instance of a general cognitive tendency to attempt to resolve ambiguities rapidly whether for linguistic . . . or perceptual input (Christiansen & Chater 2016, p. 53). Finally, pragmatic constraints must have wielded a hefty influence on many aspects of language design—Levinson (2000) showed that discourse and anaphora appear to be related, so it is plausible that aspects of binding theory could be accounted for in terms of pragmatics. In all these ways, and without doubt very many more (including ways yet to be explored—a monumental undertaking, really), language has been "shaped by the brain," naturally and parsimoniously explaining the child's relative ease of acquisition and the intimate relationship between the child's innate endowment and the structure of language.

Before concluding this section, I should indicate something of the process of mutual fit and accommodation as it occurs in the other direction. While language has been predominantly shaped by the brain, to be sure, in certain limited respects it is at least likely that the *brain* has been shaped through selection pressures *for language*. In the previous section, I mentioned that in order for adaptations to arise, evolution requires a stable environment, and that adaptations for language specifically would require a linguistically stable environment. I also said that linguistic and other cultural environments are in the nature of things quite unstable, and that given these contingencies, when it comes to cultural environments, plasticity is typically favored over robustness. This is just to say that unstable environments are conducive to the sorts of nervous systems that exploit the same resources for alternative ends, so that the cognitive mechanisms that are selected for in such circumstances will typically be flexible enough to be put to alternative uses (Avital & Jablonka 2000; Dor & Jablonka 2010). Now is as good a time as any to reference the well-known phenomenon of "niche construction," part of the "Extended Synthesis" in evolutionary biology (see Laland et al. 2015 and Laland et al. 2011 for reviews). Niche construction is a specific instance of the broader process of gene–culture coevolution (Boyd et al. 2011; Richerson & Boyd 2005). The essential difference is that the process is cumulative. Organisms are always altering their environments to better suit their needs, whether by creating nests, burrows, or dams, and so on. In the case of humans, these environmental modifications extend to the social and cultural worlds that encompass language. The changes wrought in these ways inevitably modify the selection pressures acting on organisms and so facilitate adaptation to the new environments they have created, which organisms will inevitably alter further still, which leads to new selection pressures, and so on and on in a virtuous cycle of organism-directed environmental and cultural modification and adaption that results in organisms' being increasingly better adapted to the material, social, and cultural worlds of their own making. It is highly likely that cognitive mechanisms evolved for language in this manner (*not* ELUs, however: see next paragraph), particularly to the extent that we can identify universal, stable features across linguistic environments (such as a constrained range of phonemic units arranged combinatorically and with duality of patterning). Laland (2016, p. 5) conjectures that "[i]mportant elements of infant-directed speech, such as infants' sensitivity to its linguistic features, or adults' tendency to engage in behaviour that elicits rewarding responses from infants (e.g., smiles), have been favoured through a biological evolutionary process." Adding to the list of adaptations that would have been crucial in the evolution of a language faculty, we could cite the ability to represent symbolically (Deacon 1997), the ability to reason about other minds (Malle 2002), the ability to engage in pragmatics (Levinson 2000), increased working memory (Gruber 2002), an increased domain-general capacity for learning words (Bloom 2000), and modifications to the human vocal tract (descended larynx, etc.) (de Boer 2016).

It is vital to stress that in respect of none of these adaptations can we say that we are we dealing with an ELU—language may have provided the occasion for selection, but there is no evidence that these mechanisms are used exclusively for language, and indeed *overwhelming* evidence that the brain simply "doesn't work that way": virtually no cortical structure, not even the visual cortex(!), is so insensitive to experience that it resists all cooption during development. Rather, the evidence points to a brain that integrates all sorts of brain regions within the neural ecology for the management of organism–environment interactions, even where these regions might by nature be disposed to processing particular sorts of inputs over others. This makes good evolutionary sense, being overall "a more efficient use of metabolically expensive brain matter" (Anderson 2014, p. 46). Even the structure of the vocal apparatus has uses outside the language faculty (in music and meditation, for example).

One last thing: cognitive adaptations relevant to a specific domain like language may require no more than a simple change to synaptic connection patterns; for instance, a genetic event that entrenches a pattern of connections between a set of preexisting domain-general modules (Ramus & Fisher 2009, p. 865). This is in fact just what the theory of reuse entails, at least for many cases involving the emergence of novel traits—to the extent that the theory holds that it will often be easier to mix and match existing elements than to have to evolve them afresh each time a new evolutionary challenge arises, the theory implies that specific combinations of neural elements (which have perhaps proved their value developmentally) will be selected for. How else can a specific arrangement of preexisting domain-general modules be entrenched other than through a robust synaptogenetic process of some description or another (see § 7.5 on "search")? Thus it could be that some parts of the language C-network, perhaps even large parts, are already wired up and ready to go, even though the modules within the network are entirely domain-general. Preformed connections would surely result in a smooth period of language learning, even given "relatively slight exposure and without specific training" (Chomsky 1975, p. 4).

7.5 Accounting for Linguistic Modularization

Throughout this chapter, I have been investigating a very particular question, and an important one: Does language rely on specialized cognitive and neural machinery, or does it rely on the same machinery that allows us to get by in other domains of human endeavor? The question is bound up with many other questions of no less importance: questions concerning the uniqueness of the human mind, the course of biological evolution, and the power of human culture. What is perhaps a little unusual about this question, however—unusual for a question whose answer concerns those working in both the sciences and the humanities—is that it can be phrased as a polar interrogative; i.e., as a question that admits of a yes or no response. And indeed the question has divided psychologists, linguists, and the cognitive science community generally for many decades now, more or less into two camps. In this concluding section, I would like to sketch the beginnings of an answer to this question in a way that does not pretend it can receive a simple yes or no answer. Let me stress again that neural reuse is undeniable, that the evidence for it is simply overwhelming, and that it has left no domain of psychology untouched. There seems to be nothing so specialized in the cortex that it cannot be repurposed to meet new challenges. In that regard, to be sure, what I am proposing in this section is unapologetically on the side of those who maintain that language is *not* special—that there is no specialized "language organ" or ELU. And yet I would like to carefully distinguish this claim from the claim that there are no areas of the brain that subserve exclusively linguistic functions. The neuropsychological literature offers striking examples of what appear to be fairly clean dissociations between linguistic and nonlinguistic capacities; i.e., cases in which language-processing capacities appear to be disrupted without impeding other cognitive abilities, and cases in which the reverse situation holds (Fedorenko et al. 2011; Hickok & Poeppel 2000; Poeppel 2001; Varley et al. 2005; Luria et al. 1965; Peretz & Coltheart 2003; Apperly et al. 2006). An example would be where the ability to hear words is disrupted, but the ability to recognize non-word sounds is spared (Hickok & Poeppel 2000; Poeppel 2001). Discussing such cases, Pinker and Jackendoff (2005, p. 207) add that "[c]ases of amusia and auditory agnosia, in which patients can understand speech yet fail to appreciate music or recognize environmental sounds . . . show that speech and non-speech perception in fact doubly dissociate." Although, as we saw in Chapter 4, dissociations are compatible with reuse—indeed, there is work suggesting that focal lesions can produce specific cognitive impairments within a range of non-classical architectures (Plaut 1995)—and it is equally true that often the dissociations reported are noisy (Cowie 2008, at § 3.6.3), still, their very ubiquity needs to be taken seriously and accounted for in a more systematic fashion than many defenders of reuse have been willing to do (see, e.g., Anderson 2010, p. 248, 2014, pp. 46–48). After all, a good deal of support for theories of reuse comes from the neuroimaging literature, which, as I have pointed out several times already, is somewhat ambiguous taken by itself. As Fedorenko et al. (2011, p. 16428) explain:

> standard functional MRI group analysis methods can be deceptive: two different mental functions that activate neighbouring but non-overlapping cortical regions in every subject individually can produce overlapping activations in a group analysis, because the precise locations of these regions vary across subjects, smearing the group activations. Definitively addressing the question of neural overlap between linguistic and nonlinguistic functions requires examining overlap within individual subjects, a data analysis strategy that has almost never been applied in neuroimaging investigations of high-level linguistic processing.

When Fedorenko and her colleagues applied this strategy themselves, they found that "most of the key cortical regions engaged in high-level linguistic processing are not engaged by mental arithmetic, general working memory, cognitive control or musical processing," and they think that this indicates "a high degree of functional specificity in the brain regions that support language" (2011, p. 16431). While I do not believe that claims of this strength have the least warrant—as I shall explain, functional specificity cannot be established merely by demonstrating that a region is selectively engaged by a task—these results do at least substantiate the dissociation literature in an interesting way and make it more difficult for those who would prefer to dismiss the dissociations with a ready-made list of alternative explanations. Similar results were found by Fedorenko et al. (2012).

I think neural redundancy is the best explanation for what we see in cases like these, and that redundancy is in fact a central feature of cortical design. As I briefly mentioned in Chapter 6, the brain incorporates a large measure of redundancy of function (Edelman & Gally 2001; Mason 2010; Whiteacre 2010; Deacon 2010; Iriki & Taoka 2012; Maleszka et al. 2013). Modules (M-networks) and similar structures in the brain fall into an iterative, repetitive, and almost lattice-like arrangement in the cortex. Neighboring modules have similar response properties: laminar and columnar changes are for the most part smooth—not abrupt—as one moves across the cortex, and adjacent modules do not differ markedly from one another in their basic structure and computations (if they even differ at all when taken in such proximity). Regional *solitarity* is therefore not likely to be a characteristic of the brain (Anderson 2014, p. 141).[10] We do not, in all likelihood, have just one module for X and one module for Y, but in effect several copies of the module for X and several copies of the module for Y, all densely stuffed into the same cortical zones. As Buxhoeveden and Casanova (2002, p. 943) explain of neurons generally:

> In the cortex, more cells do the job that fewer do in other regions. . . . As brain evolution paralleled the increase in cell number, a reduction occurred in the sovereignty of individual neurones; fewer of them occupy critical positions. As a consequence, plasticity and redundancy have increased. In nervous systems containing only a few hundred thousand neurones, each cell plays a more essential role in the function of the organism than systems containing billions of neurones.

[10] The term "solitarity" is Anderson's, but while he concedes that solitarity will be "relatively rare," he does not appear to believe that anything particularly significant follows from this. See also Anderson (2010, p. 296).

The same principle very likely holds true for functionally distinct groupings of neurons (i.e., modules), as Jungé and Dennett conjecture:

> It is possible that specialized brain areas contain a large amount of structural/computational redundancy (i.e., many neurons or collections of neurons that can potentially perform the same class of functions). Rather than a single neuron or small neural tract playing roles in many high-level processes, it is possible that distinct subsets of neurons within a specialized area have similar competencies, and hence are redundant, but as a result are available to be assigned individually to specific uses. . . . In a coarse enough grain, this neural model would look exactly like multi-use (or reuse). (2010, p. 278)

This is plausibly why capacities that are functionally very closely related, but for whatever reason are forced to recruit different neural circuits, will often be localized in broadly the same regions of the brain. For instance, first and second languages acquired early in ontogeny settle down in nearly the same region of Broca's area; and even when the second language is acquired in adulthood, the second language is still represented within Broca's area (while artificial languages are not) (Kandel & Hudspeth 2013). The neural coactivation graphs of such C-networks must look very similar. Indeed these results suggest—and a Redundancy Model would predict—that two very similar tasks that for whatever reason are forced to recruit different neural circuits should exhibit similar patterns of activation.

The significance of this simple but surprisingly neglected feature of cortical design cannot be overstated. Indeed, I think it should rank alongside reuse as an organizing principle of the brain, for what it actually *means* for reuse is quite interesting. Although there is abundant evidence of the reuse of the same neural *tokens* to accomplish different tasks (see Chapters 3 and 5), redundancy means we must accept that at least some of the time what we will really be witnessing is reuse of the same *types* to accomplish these tasks.[11] To my mind, this does not in any way diminish the standing of reuse. To the extent that a particular composite reuses types, and is dissociable *pro tanto*—residing in segregated brain tissue that is not active outside the function concerned—it is true that to that extent its constituents will *appear* to be

---

[11] For a developmental twist on the type/token distinction invoked in the context of modular theorizing about the mind, see Barrett (2006).

domain-specific. But in this case looks will be deceiving. The classical under-standing of domain specificity in effect *assumes* solitarity—that a module for X does something that no other module can do as well, or that *even if* another module can do X as well, taken together, these X-ing modules do not per-form outside the X-domain. Here is an example of the latter idea (Bergeron 2007, p. 176):

> a pocket calculator could have four different division modules, one for di-viding numbers smaller than or equal to 99 by numbers smaller than or equal to 99, a second one for dividing numbers smaller than or equal to 99 by numbers greater than 99, a third one for dividing numbers greater than 99 by numbers greater than 99, and a fourth one for dividing numbers greater than 99 by numbers smaller than or equal to 99. In such a calculator, these four capacities could all depend on (four versions of) the same algo-rithm. Yet, random damage to one or more of these modules in a number of such calculators could lead to observable (double) dissociations between any two of these functions.

Here, each module performs fundamentally the same algorithm, but in distinct hardware, such that dissociations are observable between any two functions. Notice, however, that none of these modules performs outside the "division" domain. This is what allows such duplicate modules to be consid-ered domain-specific—they perform functions that, for all that they might run in parallel on duplicate hardware, are unique to a specific domain of op-eration; in this case, division. If such modules could do work outside the divi-sion domain, they would lose the status of domain specificity, and acquire the status of domain neutrality (i.e., they would be domain-general). This is why a module that appears dedicated to a particular function may not be domain-specific in the classical sense. Dedication is not the same as domain speci-ficity, and redundancy, whether of calculator algorithms or neural circuits, explains why. A composite will be dedicated without being domain-specific if its functional resources are accessible to other domains through the de-ployment (reuse) of neural surrogates (i.e., redundant or "proxy" tokens). In this case, its constituents will be multi-potential but single-use (Jungé & Dennett 2010, p. 278), and the domain specificity on display somewhat cosmetic. In other words, the elements here will *look* like type B modules, but in essence they are type C modules (or even type D regions). To take an example with more immediate relevance to the brain, a set of modules that are structurally and computationally similar may be equally suited for face-recognition tasks, abstract-object-recognition tasks, the recognition of moving objects, and so on. One of these modules could be reserved for faces, another for abstract objects, another for moving objects, and so on. What is noteworthy is that, while the functional activation may be indistinguishable in each case, and the same type of resource will be employed on each occasion, a *different* token module will be at work at any one time. To quote Jungé and Dennett again: "In an adult brain, a given neuron [or set of neurons] would be aligned with only a single high-level function, whereas each area of neurons would be aligned with very many different functions" (2010, p. 278). Such modules (and composites) are for all intents and purposes *qualitatively* identical, though clearly not *numerically* identical, meaning that, while they share their properties, they are not *one and the same* (Parfit 1984). The evidence of reuse is virtually all one way when it comes to the pervasiveness of functional inheritance across cognitive domains. It may be that this inheritance owes to reuse of the same tokens (literal reuse) or to reuse of the same types (reuse by proxy), but the inheritance itself has been amply attested. This broader notion of reuse still offers a crucial insight into the operations of cognition, and I daresay represents a large part of the appeal of the original massive redeployment hypothesis (Anderson 2007c).

It is interesting to note in this respect that, although detractors have frequently pointed out the ambiguity of neuroimaging evidence on account of its allegedly coarse spatial resolution (see § 3.3.3), suggesting that the same area will be active across separate tasks even if distinct but adjacent circuits are involved each time, this complaint can have no bearing whatsoever on reuse by proxy. Fedorenko et al. (2011, p. 16431) take their neuroimaging evidence to support "a high degree of functional specificity in the brain regions that support language," but their results do not license this extreme claim. The regions they found to have been selectively engaged by linguistic tasks were all adjacent to the regions engaged in nonlinguistic tasks. Elementary considerations suggest that they have discovered a case of reuse by proxy involving language: the domains tested (mental arithmetic, general working memory, cognitive control, and musical processing) make use of many of the same computations as high-level linguistic processing, even though they run them on duplicate hardware. Redundancy makes it is easy to see how fairly sharp dissociations could arise—knocking out one token module need disrupt only one high-level operation: other high-level operations that draw on the same type of resource may well be spared.

The consequences of this distinction between literal reuse and reuse by proxy for much speculation about the localization and specialization of function are potentially profound. In cognitive neuropsychology, the discovery that a focal lesion selectively impairs a particular cognitive function is routinely taken as evidence of its functional specificity (Coltheart 2011; Sternberg 2011). Even cognitive scientists who take a developmental approach to modularity—i.e., who concede that parts of the mind may be modular but stress that modularization is a developmental process—concede too much when they imply, as they frequently do, that modularization results in domain-specific modules (Karmiloff-Smith 1992; Prinz 2006; Barrett 2006; Cowie 2008; Guida et al. 2016). This is true in some sense, but not in anything like the standard sense, for the Redundancy Model envisages that developmental modules form a special class of C-networks; namely, those that are *qualitatively* identical but *numerically* distinct. The appearance of modularization in development is thus fully compatible with deep domain interpenetration. In any event, the Redundancy Model does not predict that all acquired skills will be modular. The evidence suggests that, while some complex skills reside in at least partly dissociable circuitry, most complex skills are implemented in more typical C-networks (i.e., those consisting of literally shared parts).[12]

In one sense, asking why the cortex incorporates a large measure of redundancy of function is a bit like asking why we have two eyes, two kidneys, ten toes, and so on. The intuitive response is that by having "spare" organs, we can distribute the workload more efficiently among all of them. It is generally a good design feature of any system to have spare capacity. For instance, in engineered systems, "redundant parts can substitute for others that malfunction or fail, or augment output when demand for a particular output increases" (Whiteacre 2010, 14). The positive connection between robustness and redundancy in biological systems is clear (Edelman and Gally 2001; Mason 2010; Whiteacre 2010; Iriki & Taoka 2012). So there are good reasons for evolution to have seen to it that our brains have spare capacity. But in the case of the brain and the cortex most especially, there are other reasons why redundancy would be an important design feature. It offers a solution to what Jungé and Dennett (2010, p. 278) called the "time-sharing" problem. It may also offer a solution to what I call the "encapsulation" problem.

---

[12] This seems to be true regardless of whether the complex skills are innate or acquired.

The time-sharing problem arises when multiple simultaneous demands are made on the same cognitive resource. This is probably a regular occurrence, and language in particular would present a whole host of opportunities for time-sharing. Here are just a few examples.

- Driving a car and holding a conversation at the same time: if it is true that some of the selfsame motor operations underlying aspects of speech production and comprehension are also required for the execution of sequenced or complex motor functions (as is perhaps exemplified by driving a manual vehicle, or operating complex machinery), how do we manage to pull this off?
- By reflecting the recursive structure of thought, the coding function may redeploy the recursive operation simultaneously during sentence production. This might be the case during the formation of an embedded relative clause—the thought and its encoding may require parallel use of the same sequencing principle. Again, how do we manage this feat?
- If metarepresentational operations are involved in the internalization of conventional sound–meaning pairs, and also in the pragmatics and mindreading that carry on simultaneously during conversation, as argued by Suddendorf (2013), it could be another instance of time-sharing. The example is contentious, but it still raises the question: How does our brain manage to do things like this?
- Christiansen and Chater's (2016) "Chunk and Pass" model of language processing envisages *multilevel* and *simultaneous* chunking procedures. As they put it, "the challenge of language acquisition is to learn a dazzling sequence of rapid processing operations" (2016, p. 116). What must the brain be like to allow for this dazzling display?

Explaining these phenomena is difficult. Indeed, when dealing with clear (literal) instances of reuse, results from the interference paradigm show that processing bottlenecks are inevitable—true multitasking is impossible (see § 4.2.3). Redundancy offers a natural explanation of how the brain overcomes the time-sharing problem. It explains, in short, how we are able to "walk and chew gum" at the same time.

Redundancy might also offer a solution to the encapsulation problem. As I explained in § 4.2.3, functional composites are not likely to be characterized by informational encapsulation, because in sharing their parts with other systems they will prima facie have access to the information stored and manipulated by those other systems (Anderson 2010, p. 300). If overlapping brain networks must share information on some level (Pessoa 2016, p. 23), it would be reasonable to suppose that central and peripheral systems do not overlap. This is because peripheral systems, which are paradigmatically fast and automatic, would not be able to process inputs as efficiently if there were a serious risk of central system override—i.e., of beliefs and other central information getting in the way of automatic processing. But we know from the neuroimaging literature that quite often the brain networks implementing central and peripheral functions do overlap. This is puzzling in light of the degree of cognitive impenetrability that certain sensory systems still seem to exhibit—limited though it may be. If it is plausible to suppose that the phenomenon calls for segregated circuitry, redundancy could feature in a solution to the puzzle, since it naturally explains how the brain can make parallel use of the same resources. Neuroimaging maps might well display what appear to be overlapping brain regions between two tasks (one involving central information, the other involving classically peripheral operations), but the overlap would not exist—there would be distinct, albeit adjacent and nearly identical, circuits recruited in each case. Of course, there may be other ways around the encapsulation problem that do not require segregated circuitry: the nature and extent of the overlap is presumably important. But clearly, redundancy opens up some fascinating explanatory possibilities.

To the extent that acquired skills must overcome both the time-sharing problem as well as the encapsulation problem—for acquired competencies are often able to run autonomously of central processes—we might expect that their neural implementations incorporate redundant tissue. In concluding, let me illustrate this point by offering a gloss on a particular account of how skills and expertise are acquired during development elaborated by Guida et al. (2016) and Anderson (2014). The process involved is called "search." Search is an exploratory synaptogenetic process, "the active testing of multiple neuronal combinations until finding the most appropriate one for a specific skill, i.e., the neural niche of that skill" (Guida et al. 2016, p. 13). The theory holds that, in the early stages of skill acquisition, the brain must search for an appropriate mix of brain areas and does so by recruiting relatively widely across the cortex. When expertise has finally developed, a much narrower and more specific network of brain areas has been settled upon, such that "[a]s a consequence of their extended practice, experts develop domain-specific knowledge structures" (Guida et al. 2016, p. 13). The gloss (and my hunch) is this: first, that repeated practice of a task that requires segregation (to get around time-sharing and encapsulation issues) will in effect *force* search into redundant neural terrain (Karmiloff-Smith 1992; Barrett 2006; Barrett & Kurzban 2006); second, that search will recruit idle or relatively underutilized circuits in preference to busy ones as a general default strategy. Guida et al. (2016) cite evidence that experts' brains reuse areas of which novices' brains make only limited use: "novices use episodic long-term memory areas (e.g., the mediotemporal lobe) for performing long-term memory tasks," but "experts are able to (re)use these areas also for performing working-memory tasks" (Guida et al. 2016, p. 14). Guida et al., in agreement with Anderson (2014), seem to have literal reuse in mind. But the same evidence they cite is consistent with reuse by proxy. As Barrett and Kurzban (2006, p. 639) suggest, echoing a similar suggestion by Karmiloff-Smith (1992), a developmental system

> could contain a procedure or mechanism that partitioned off certain tasks— shunting them into a dedicated developmental pathway—under certain conditions, for example, when the cue structure of repeated instances of the task clustered tightly together, and when it was encountered repeatedly, as when highly practiced. . . . Under this scenario, reading could still be recruiting an evolved system for object recognition, and yet phenotypically there could be distinct modules for reading and for other types of object recognition.

7.6 Summary

In any reasonable construal of the language faculty, language is not cognitively special vis-à-vis other cognitive domains. There seems to be no language module, no elementary linguistic unit, no hardwired language organ. Language was likely to have been assembled from older sensory-motor and nonlinguistic materials. Neuroimaging, biobehavioral, computational, and evolutionary considerations all point to the same conclusion. Such linguistic adaptations as there have been have been coopted in many other domains of cognition. The sort of cultural environment in which language consists is too unstable to provide the conditions for typical selection scenarios in which robust phenotypes can emerge, and the brain anyway negotiates energetic constraints by repurposing existing resources to meet new challenges. Language acquisition frequently does seem effortless on the child's part and exhibits a degree of developmental robustness. But the ease of acquisition has probably been exaggerated, and the child's environment is not so impoverished as was once assumed. In any case, such ease of acquisition can be explained in other ways than by postulating exotic and impossible-to-evolve circuitry. Language has been shaped by the brain far more than the brain has been shaped by language. Cultural evolution is a powerful factor in human history and is more than sufficient to explain why languages seem to run so well with the grain of the human mind. It is true that language dissociates from other cognitive skills, at least in some respects, but the Redundancy Model puts this sort of modularization in its proper context. The Redundancy Model predicates functional inheritance across tasks and task categories, even when the tasks are implemented in spatially segregated neural networks. Thus dissociation evidence alone does not always indicate functional specificity. In particular, these dissociations provide no evidence that language is cognitively special.

8

Saving Faculty Psychology

Debunking the Argument from Multiple Realization

8.1 New Directions in Faculty Psychology

The discovery that traditional psychological faculties are implemented by neural systems consisting of shared domain-general components does not make traditional faculty psychology go away. On the contrary, as I argued in § 4.2.3, these high-level cognitive systems—I decline to call them modules—have an important role to play in our ongoing quest to understand the mind. The ramifications of reuse will in fact serve to sharpen our understanding of what makes these systems tick and reveal the extent of functional and semantic inheritance between traditional tasks and task categories. A mature twenty-first-century faculty psychology, therefore, has a lot to look forward to—and essentially nothing to fear. But if the work required to understand behavior in the light of neural reuse is going to get done by anyone, it will have to get done (one would think, in the first instance at least) by twenty-first-century faculty psychologists! All those with a wealth of experience investigating the higher faculties will simply have to get on board if the endeavor is to have any chance of success. In other words, the future of faculty psychology depends in no small part on the productive collaboration between neuroscience and psychology.

Unfortunately, there is a potential obstruction in the way of just this sort of intertheoretic collaboration. Inasmuch as high-level cognitive systems are understood to be software systems, pitched at the level of algorithmic or computational psychology, the thought arises that these systems can be investigated with a kind of disciplinary immunity from neuroscience, since (it is supposed) "[n]o amount of knowledge about the hardware of a computer will tell you anything serious about the nature of the software that computer runs" (Coltheart 2004, p. 22). The idea proceeds at least

The Adaptable Mind. John Zerilli, Oxford University Press (2021). © Oxford University Press.
DOI: 10.1093/oso/9780190067885.003.0008

in part from the assumption that psychological processes are multiply realized. The multiple realization (MR) hypothesis asserts, at its baldest, that the same psychological state may be realized in neuroscientifically distinct substrates (Polger 2009). Hilary Putnam's (1967) ingenious suggestion that "pain" is likely to be a multiply realized kind (MR kind) rather neatly captures the thought here—while presumably both mammals and mollusks experience pain, they pretty obviously lack the same neurobiological basis. MR was played against a popular philosophical theory of mind in the 1960s that attempted to identify mental states with neural states. Since MR implies a many-to-one mapping from neural states to mental states, if it is in fact true that mental states are multiply realized, it follows that no clear identity relationship can hold between them. Thus it was that many of those who advanced MR rejected mind–brain identity as a viable philosophical theory. As Bechtel and Mundale (1999, p. 176) framed the issue, "[o]ne corollary of this rejection of the identity thesis is the contention that information about the brain is of little or no relevance to understanding psychological processes." Fodor et al. (1974, p. xiv) are blunt: "it is not only far from clear that neurology provides a useful theoretical vocabulary for psychology, it is even unclear that neurological theories will *ever* have much practical implication for the development of psychological models."

Another development of the argument asserts that even if MR does not hold true among existing biological systems, the possibility that cognitive states might be shared by built artifacts or alien life forms having very different physical structures in itself establishes the salience of the MR thesis. This version of the argument led some philosophers of artificial intelligence (AI) to embrace the further metaphysical claim that "mental processes are the operations themselves, and are not identified with whatever biological or other substances realize them" (Bechtel & Mundale 1999, p. 176). Following Bechtel and Mundale's lead, and the contours of the recent debate surrounding MR, I shall not address this version of the argument or the metaphysical claim it inspired here. The possibility that artifacts could have mental states is just the possibility that the identity theory is wrong, which is precisely the claim in dispute (Polger 2009, p. 459). Instead, I shall use this chapter to consider, admittedly quite briefly, the empirical claim—that the MR hypothesis can be verified having regard to existing organisms—since no doubt it is this claim that has played the lion's share in encouraging a downbeat attitude to evidence from neuroscience in some quarters.

Daniel Dennett (1991, pp. 254, 270, n. 2), for instance, laments the functionalist's penchant for "boxology"; i.e., drawing diagrams that install component functions in separate boxes, "while explicitly denying that these boxes have anatomical significance." While he concedes that "in principle" it may be a good tactic, and one he himself has employed, "it does tend to blind the functionalist to alternative decompositions of function, and particularly to the prospect of [neural reuse]." Small wonder, then, that he calls for a "better vision, anchored in a positive acceptance—as opposed to a hysterical dismissal—of the foundational facts of functional neuroanatomy" (see also McGeer 2007; Hardcastle & Stewart 2009, p. 194; Karmiloff-Smith 1994, p. 702; Bechtel 2008a, p. 990; Gerrans 2014, pp. 22–23). In § 8.2, I put the two primary empirical arguments in favor of MR under pressure, as well as offer a survey of recent arguments skeptical of the MR hypothesis.

But let me be clear at the outset. My position is in no way hostage to the fortunes of MR, however one cares to define it. There are other ways to argue for the pertinence of neuroscience to psychology that need not presuppose type identity among cognitive and neural states. I can think of at least three. For one thing, it does not pay to have an uncompromisingly rigid understanding of the reduction relationship. John Bickle (2010, pp. 250–251; 1998, p. 30) appeals to examples of successful reduction from the history of science that happened to involve MR kinds as among the posits of the reduced theories, including examples of reduction involving *radical* MR—that over distinct physical states occurring within the *same* token physical system at different times. The reduction of temperature to mean molecular kinetic energy could be considered to involve radical MR, since classical thermodynamic kinds like temperature are in truth macroscopic states multiply realized over different microstates of the same macroscopic system over time. Yet the reduction of classical thermodynamics to the kinetic/corpuscular theory of matter is "the textbook example of scientific intertheoretic reduction." In another vein, Jaegwon Kim (1992), Larry Shapiro (2000), and Colin Klein (2008) have each drawn attention to a significant dilemma confronting the MR advocate. If a given functional kind is not multiply realized, the traditional argument for its autonomy and irreducibility falls away. If, on the other hand, the kind *is* multiply realized, the kind will not be a proper scientific kind; i.e., of the sort that can enter into laws. "Brittleness" might be a multiply realized property, but glass, steel, and biscuits are each brittle in their own way: there can be no general science of brittle things. Ranging over such genuinely diverse physical realizations means the kind will not enter into laws (i.e., exhibit lawlike or projectable properties), except for those that are true analytically—such as *All mousetraps catch mice*, and *All eyes see*—and this in turn "undercut[s] the traditional motivation for admitting functional kinds into the ontologies of the special sciences" (Shapiro 2000, p. 637). Thus, if mental states really are multiply realized, neuroscience will matter very much indeed—not so much because psychology could not do without it, but because psychology's claim to be a traditional science would be open to question. This is only the most skeptical conclusion one could draw, but the point is well taken (see Couch 2009, pp. 262–264, for criticisms, however). Finally, and somewhat trivially, *multiply* realizable does not mean *infinitely* realizable. Cognitive hypotheses will always have implications for realizers—mousetraps cannot be made of paper after all. A functionalist psychology, this is to say, can proceed only within the biophysical limits that its own constructs impose, and it ignores evidence of implementation to its peril. Take modularity as an example. A commitment to modularity standardly entails a belief in the functional dissociability of at least some cognitive capacities; but this, as we saw in Chapters 4, 5, and 7, is just not the sort of feature that the evidence of reuse makes available, at any rate in a straightforward manner. Of course, neural hypotheses may themselves be disconfirmed by evidence coming from other branches of the cognitive sciences, including psychology, so the constraints here are genuinely bidirectional and intertheoretic. But MR or not, there is simply no way of getting around the neuroscience (McGeer 2007).

Be that as it may, given the recent tide of empirical challenges to the MR thesis, and because MR has proven itself to be an occasional stumbling block in the path of those committed to the autonomy of the special sciences, I have considered it worthwhile saying at least something on the subject. While the more austere school of functionalism admittedly no longer enjoys the following it once had—and mainstream functionalists today would hardly dismiss neuroscience on the basis of psychology's autonomy of neuroscience—pockets of the austere school do survive under the guise of cognitive neuropsychology and related fields (see McGeer 2007 for detailed analysis and criticism).

8.2 Multiple Realization Revisited

8.2.1 Preliminary remarks

Two primary empirical arguments have been advanced at one time or another in support of the view that cognitive states are multiply realized. One argument proceeds from evidence of extensive neuroplasticity in the brain. The other proceeds from an account of convergent evolution. In the first part of this section, I shall briefly address these arguments for MR and the existence of MR kinds. In the second part, I provide a conspectus of the most forceful arguments against MR developed in recent years.

8.2.2 Empirical arguments for multiple realization

8.2.2.1 *Neuroplasticity*

Neuroplasticity has in recent times been thought to provide compelling evidence for the MR of mental states. Shapiro (2004) and Polger (2009) review this evidence and find that it does not provide evidence of MR. Polger (2009, p. 470) concludes that "contrary to philosophical consensus, the identity theory does not blatantly fly in the face of what is known about the correlations between psychological and neural processing."

As we saw in Chapter 2, there is more than one kind of brain plasticity, including, *inter alia,* cortical map plasticity and synaptic plasticity. Very roughly, the former occurs when different brain regions subserve the same function at different times in an individual's history—say, after brain injury or trauma—and it is this plasticity that is most often regarded as supporting MR. "Synaptic plasticity" refers to the strengthening or weakening of connections between neurons, and it is believed to have a role in learning and memory (and quite possibly, therefore, in cortical map plasticity). I shall restrict myself to the first kind here.

Evidence supporting a modest identity relationship between psychology and neuroscience includes the following (Polger 2009, pp. 467–468):

- Cortical maps do not migrate wildly; i.e., they do not simply "'jump' to recruit unused but non-adjacent cortical areas," and when they appear to do so, it is generally to exploit the structural features common to different sites (see, e.g., the discussion of EB in Chapter 6).

- Recovered functions are frequently suboptimal—genuine MR would require the *same* psychological state to be underwritten by different neurological states; suboptimality is evidence that the psychological states are in fact different, and therefore evidence of difference underlying difference, not difference underlying sameness, as MR requires.[1]
- Functional studies of the rewired ferrets whose visual cortex was induced to project into auditory cortex suggest they "developed processing structures—in particular, columnar organization—that is [*sic*] typical of visual processing" within auditory cortex. Since auditory cortex came to resemble visual cortex (Shapiro 2008, p. 518), this is not evidence that auditory regions learned to handle visual domain tasks while still in their auditory configuration, as genuine MR would require here. After all, auditory regions have specific neural configurations and connection patterns. If these are not preserved when the ferret's auditory cortex begins processing visual input, it cannot be a case of MR. What we have is a case of sameness underlying sameness, not difference underlying sameness, as MR requires. Put another way, the studies are reporting a genuine case of *crossmodal* plasticity (or perhaps supramodal plasticity), not MR (see §§ 2.4.2–2.4.3).

In fact, it is unsurprising that neuroplasticity has not been able to deliver up the expected argosy of empirical support for MR, and this for two reasons. Firstly, many of the most sophisticated brain-imaging techniques to date have not been able to yield high-resolution mappings of the neural configurations implicated in rehabilitation after injury. Neither positron emission tomography (PET) nor fMRI measures neural activity and network configuration directly. What they measure, in fact, is blood flow, which can hardly tell us much about whether the functions in question are multiply realized. Even if MR were pervasive, these methods would not yield coherent, interpretable results. Why, then, assume that a recovered function with a new location should have a different realization basis, unless of course there is some other indication that makes it likely (e.g., simultaneous preservation of the old and recovered function in the new area)? Secondly, without standardized criteria for evaluating sameness/difference judgments, how can we be sure

---

[1] Actually, this argument requires care. It only goes through if it can be shown that there is a distinct *function* served by the two psychological states. I address the matter at some length in Zerilli (2019).

that neuroplasticity even speaks to MR? I conveniently neglected this consideration when making the preceding points, and in fact it is only in recent years that more careful attention has been paid to questions of sameness and difference in debates about MR. I take this up in § 8.2.3.4.

8.2.2.2 *Convergent evolution*

Evolutionary considerations, particularly the idea that convergent evolution is likely to generate psychological similarities *as well as* behavioral similarities (such as flight in birds and bats) in morphologically unrelated species, have been thought to weigh in favor of MR. But the issue cannot be decided a priori. MR is an empirical hypothesis in the end and must sooner or later come to terms with empirical evidence. In fact, evolutionary considerations might actually tell against MR. Here I cite only one case, detailed at greater length in Bickle (2003, 2010). The process by which short-term memory becomes long-term memory is known as "memory consolidation," and Bickle cites evidence supporting the likelihood of there being shared molecular mechanisms for memory consolidation across biological taxa as diverse as fruit flies, sea slugs, and mice. One might not think this sort of evidence admits of any far-reaching consequences for human psychology or MR generally, but if the instance is seen to follow from certain "core principles of molecular evolution," it assumes a larger significance. One such principle holds that the amino acid sequences of specific proteins in functionally important, "constrained," domains change much more slowly than in functionally less important domains. This principle implies the existence of "universally conserved" molecular mechanisms across distantly related biological species, albeit those found deep down in cellular physiology and intracellular signaling pathways, just as the fly/slug/mouse pathway attests.

> In the end, any psychological kind that affects an organism's behavior must involve the cell-metabolic machinery in individual neurons. In the brain, causally speaking, that's where the rubber hits the road. But that's the very machinery [that] tends to be conserved evolutionarily across existing biological species. Random changes to its components, especially to amino acid sequences in its proteins' constrained domains (almost) inevitably are detrimental to an organism's survival. (Bickle 2010, p. 258)

Far from being exceptional, "molecular evolution suggests [such mechanisms] should be the rule." So at least this empirical argument, rooted in considerations of evolutionary plausibility and molecular evolution, predicts that the MR thesis is false at the molecular level, if not at the systems level (see also Hawrylycz 2015, pp. 8–9; Koch 2015, p. 26; and Zador 2015, p. 43).

8.2.3 A conspectus of recent arguments against multiple realization

8.2.3.1 *Outline of arguments*

The most powerful arguments against the MR hypothesis as presented in the recent literature include:

- the argument from comparative psychology (Bechtel & Mundale 1999);
- the argument from grains (Bechtel & Mundale 1999); and
- the argument from context (Bechtel & Mundale 1999; Shapiro 2000; Polger & Shapiro 2008; Shapiro & Polger 2012; Polger & Shapiro 2016).

8.2.3.2 *The argument from comparative psychology*

Bechtel and Mundale (1999) appeal to "neurobiological and cognitive neuroscience practice" in the hope of showing how claims that psychological states are multiply realized are unjustified. Essentially, theirs is an argument from success: cognitive neuroscience's method assumes MR is false, and the success of that method is evidence that MR *is* false. They argue that it is "precisely on the basis of working assumptions about commonalities in brains across individuals and species that neurobiologists and cognitive neuroscientists have discovered clues to the information processing being performed" (1999, p. 177).

Bechtel and Mundale examine both the "neuroanatomical and neurophysiological practice of carving up the brain." What they believe this examination reveals is, firstly, that the principle of psychological function plays an essential role in both disciplines, and secondly, that "the cartographic project itself is frequently carried out comparatively—across species" (1999, p. 177), the opposite of what one would expect if MR were "a serious option." It is the very similarity (or homology) of brain structures that permits generalization across species; and similarity in the functional characterization of homologous brain regions across species only makes sense if the claims of MR are either false or greatly exaggerated. For instance, "[e]ven with the advent of neuroimaging, permitting localization of processing areas in humans, research on brain visual areas remains fundamentally dependent on monkey research" (1999, p. 195). Brodmann's famous brain maps were based upon comparisons of altogether 55 species and 11 orders of mammals. If MR were true, "one would not expect results based on comparative neuroanatomical and neurophysiological studies to be particularly useful in developing functional accounts of human psychological processing" (1999, p. 178). They also argue that the ubiquity of brain mapping as a way of decomposing cognitive function points to the implausibility of the MR thesis. The understanding of psychological function is increasingly "being fostered by appeal to the brain and its organization" (1999, p. 191), again, the opposite of what one would expect "[i]f the taxonomies of brain states and psychological states were as independent of each other as the [MR] argument suggests" (1999, pp. 190–191).

Aizawa (2009, pp. 500–503) detects a tacit claim in Bechtel and Mundale to the effect that unique cross-species localization of functions in the brain entails their unique realization. This is thought to be a *non sequitur*. It is true that, strictly speaking, what much of their paper succeeds in showing is the unlikelihood of "multiple *localization*," but two things can be said in response. Firstly, the criticism to some extent misses the point of their analysis. Bechtel and Mundale have *deliberately* opted for functional localization; i.e., brain activity in the same parts or conglomerate of parts across species, as the relevant standard by which to judge the sameness or difference of brain states, and they have done so in deference to cognitive neuroscience practice. Localization is for them the appropriate standard to adopt because it is at the right grain of description (see next section, 8.2.3.3). Secondly, it is not actually easy to police the distinction between localization and realization, for neural localization is an important dimension of neural organization. Aizawa complains that Bechtel and Mundale do not provide independent evidence in support of any such proposition, but, all in all, it does not seem to be a particularly tendentious one.[2] It is true that, for all we know, functions could be localized in the same region in closely related species, and yet be organized very differently. But surely we would need some reason to think that this is likely.

---

[2] It only appears to be tendentious when a certain paradigm of realization and MR, the so-called dimensioned view, has one under its sway (see Gillett 2003).

A more serious criticism of their argument is that it speaks only to species that are homologous—it might demonstrate that the ubiquity of MR is questionable as long as we restrict our gaze to primates and rodents (i.e., mammals generally, related by common descent), but surely it does not succeed in showing that octopuses and humans realize their psychologies in anything like the same way (Kim 2002; Shapiro 2008). Nevertheless, the arguments grounded in methodological and comparative considerations offer an impressive refutation of MR among the many that have been attempted in the past 15 or so years. Clearly there is *some* notion of similarity at stake here that, while largely unarticulated in Bechtel and Mundale, ultimately needs to be reckoned with—at least among homologues (cf. Gillett 2002, 2003; Polger & Shapiro 2008).

Next, I present two distinct but related arguments, the argument from grains and the argument from context. Bechtel and Mundale have something to say about both, whereas Shapiro confines his analysis, as far as we shall be concerned, to the import of context alone.

8.2.3.3 *The argument from grains*

Bechtel and Mundale (1999, pp. 178–179, 201–204) resort to grains as a way of making sense of what they perceive to be the entrenched, almost unquestioning consensus prevailing around MR. They think this can be traced to the practice of philosophers' appealing to different grain sizes in the taxonomies of psychological and brain states, "using a coarse grain in lumping together psychological states and a fine grain in splitting brain states." When Putnam went about collecting his various specimens of pain, he ignored the many likely nuances between them. At the same time, he had few compunctions about declaring them different at a neurological level. His contention that pain is likely to be an MR kind can only command our respect if we can be sure that when he was comparing his specimens from a neurological point of view, he was careful to apply no less lenient a standard of differentiation than he applied when comparing his specimens from a psychological point of view. Bechtel and Mundale maintain that when "a common grain size is insisted on, as it is in scientific practice, the plausibility of multiple realizability evaporates." As their examples of neuroanatomical and neurophysiological practice attest, scientists in these fields typically match a coarse-grained conception of psychological states with an equally coarse-grained conception of brain states. Despite the habit of philosophers' individuating brain states in accordance with physical and chemical criteria, a habit no doubt originating with Putnam, this is not how neuroscientists characterize them. The notion of a brain state is "a philosopher's fiction" (1999, p. 177), given that the notion neuroscientists actually employ is much less fine-grained; namely, "activity in the same brain part or conglomerate of parts."

8.2.3.4 *The argument from context*

A not-unrelated factor that Bechtel and Mundale think might help explain the prevailing MR consensus in philosophy and the mind sciences is that the hypothesis itself is often presented in a "contextual vacuum." The choice of grain is always determined by context, with "different contexts for constructing taxonomies" resulting in "different grain sizes for both psychology and neuroscience." The development of evolutionary perspectives, for instance, in which the researcher necessarily adopts a coarse grain, contrasts with the much finer grain that will be appropriate when assessing differences among conspecifics. "One can adopt either a coarse or a fine grain, but as long as one uses a comparable grain on both the brain and mind side, the mapping between them will be correspondingly systematic."

Shapiro (2000), more alive than most to the acuteness of the metaphysical problem central to MR, has provided perhaps the most useful and philosophically perceptive treatment of sameness/difference judgments as they relate to MR. He states: "Before it is possible to evaluate the force of [the MR thesis] in arguments against reductionism, we must be in a position to say with assurance what the satisfaction conditions for [the MR thesis] actually are" (2000, p. 636). For him: "The general lesson is this. Showing that a kind is multiply realizable, or that two realizations of a kind are in fact distinct, requires some work" (2000, p. 645), and "[t]o establish [the MR thesis], one must show that the differences among purported realizations are causally relevant differences" (2000, p. 646).

Shapiro's concerns revolve around what motivates ascriptions of difference, and therefore sameness. The issue is important because the classic intuition pump that asks us to conceive of a mind in which every neuron has been replaced by a silicon chip depends on our ascription of an interesting difference between neurons and silicon chips, apparently even where silicon chips can be made that contribute to psychological capacity by one and the same process of electrical transmission. His answer, too, like Bechtel and Mundale's, depends ultimately on context—in particular, the context set by the very inquiry into MR itself.

Shapiro (2000, pp. 643–644) argues that "the things for which [the MR thesis] has a chance of being true" are all "defined by reference to their purpose or capacity or contribution to some end." This is the reason why carburetors, mousetraps, computers, and minds are standard metaphors in the literature of MR. They are defined "in virtue of what they do," unlike, say, water, which is typically defined by what it is—i.e., its constitution or molecular structure, and accordingly *not* an MR kind. Genuine MR requires that there be "*different* ways to bring about the function that defines the kind." Truly distinct (indeed *multiple*) realizations are those that "differ in causally relevant properties—in properties that make a difference to how [the realizations] contribute to the capacity under investigation." Two corkscrews differing only in color are not distinct realizations of a corkscrew, because color "makes no difference to their performance as a corkscrew." Similarly, the difference between steel and aluminum is not enough to make two corkscrews that are alike in all other respects two different realizations of a corkscrew "because, relative to the properties that make them suitable for removing corks, they are identical." In this instance, differences of composition can be "screened off." Naturally, there may be cases where differences of composition *will* be causally relevant—perhaps rigidity is the allegedly MR kind in question, in which case compositional differences will necessarily speak to how aluminum and steel achieve this disposition. Each case must simply be judged on its own merits, indeed, in its own context (as Bechtel and Mundale might put it). Thus, unlike the two corkscrews identical in all respects save color, which do not count as distinct realizations, waiters' corkscrews and winged corkscrews are enabled to perform the same task by virtue of *different* causally relevant properties, and therefore *do* count as genuinely distinct realizations of a corkscrew, one based on the principle of simple leverage, the other relying on a rack and pinions (see Fig. 8.1).

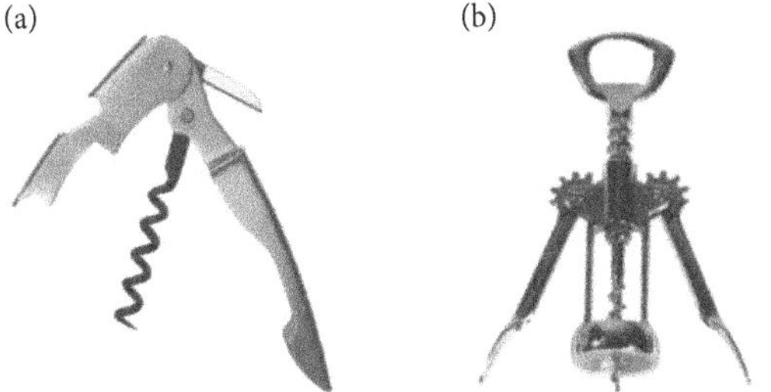

Figure 8.1   A waiter's corkscrew (a) and a winged corkscrew (b). Each contributes to the capacity of cork-removal in different ways.

The problem for the MR advocate is this: it is apparent that each of the examples just given involves a straightforward mechanism that renders its classification reasonably intuitive (though I dare say still subject to the odd disagreement!). With the brain, the situation is inestimably more complicated, so why should the MR advocate feel so confident that there is more than one *truly* distinct way to build a mind, given that we know comparatively little about how brains produce minds in the first place? One might even think that the brain's functional properties would need to be understood at least as well as the corkscrew's before one could venture an opinion about whether truly different brains can produce similar minds.[3]

8.2.4   Conclusion

The primary empirical arguments for MR resting on weak evidence at best, the functionalist has more work to do before she can, by her lights with a clean conscience, look askance at the neural evidence and its implications for cognitive theorizing.

8.3 New Look Faculty Psychology

Exactly how the science of mental faculties will have to change to accommodate the reality of neural reuse is a matter of some uncertainty, but even those such as Michael Silberstein who assert that "the autonomy and irreducibility of folk psychology are assured" concede that reuse means "scientific psychology must be heavily revised" (2016, pp. 27–28). My position, and the position it was the aim of the previous section to make feasible, is that psychology and neuroscience are friends, not enemies. I start from the premise that the best way to understand something is to break it down, and that the best and most natural way to break something down is to carve it at its joints; i.e., in such a way as to respect its physical constitution and design. I take this to be near truism. Now the fact remains that, as I have tried to show, the endeavor to understand the mind has come a long way from the days when

---

[3] Shapiro and Polger (2012, p. 282) elaborate upon Shapiro's (2000) pragmatic considerations and attempt to situate his criteria within a somewhat more formal rubric. See also Shapiro (2008, pp. 522–525), Polger (2008), Polger (2009, pp. 463–464), and Polger and Shapiro (2016).

Herbert Simon and David Marr reasoned from evolutionary principles that the carve-up of relevance to the mind produces independently modifiable subcomponents that correspond to functionally specific units of high-level psychology (Sternberg 2011, p. 158). I am not saying that the mind is bereft of dissociable subcomponents (see Chapters 4 and 5), but our ideas about them have certainly changed. As long as psychology wishes to carve nature at its joints, then, it will have to update its ideas about what those joints are. At a minimum, neural reuse mandates an approach to decomposition that assigns domain-neutral functions to brain regions; and if such regions are the stuff of higher-level cognition, it is surely not reasonable to insulate the higher-level cognitive ontology from their effects. One does not have to be a ruthless reductionist or eliminativist to recommend that our sciences so develop as to facilitate mutual interaction and even potentially unification. If this is right, cognitive models of distinct domains should be placed upon such a footing as will best accommodate the possibility of interaction. We will learn *more* about the faculties, not less, if we can appreciate their deeper-level associations. It is interesting to note in this respect that the 2010 edition of David Marr's *Vision*—a book that is (in)famous for having made the strict independence between levels of inquiry an article of faith in the cognitive sciences—contains an Afterword that chimes nicely with the message I am trying to convey here:

> (1) insights gained on higher levels help us ask the right questions and do the right experiments at the lower levels, and (2) it is necessary to study nervous systems at all levels simultaneously. From this perspective, the importance of coupling experimental and theoretical work in the neurosciences follows directly; without close interaction with experiments, theory is very likely to be sterile. (2010 [1982], p. 364)

One example of this mutual endeavor can be seen in neurolinguistic work that tries to integrate formal results from the Minimalist Program in syntax. (In adverting to this work, I do not mean to endorse the Minimalist Program, only to illustrate how researchers in fields that have typically been seen as antagonistic to one another can come together in the interests of science.) David Poeppel (2015) remarks that the goals of systems neuroscience and research in syntax have aligned in the past two decades. I touched upon some of the relevant systems neuroscience in my discussion of canonical neural computations (§ 7.3). The discovery of primitive computations such as filtering, divisive normalization, and predictive coding bodes well for the basic assumptions behind the Minimalist Program. Both research programs seek to uncover fundamental and (as much as possible) domain-general operations underlying various cognitive phenomena. Merge can be seen as another such computation (§ 7.2). The part of Merge that combines elements is a close analogue of *binding* (or *concatenation*) operations within systems neuroscience (Poeppel 2015, p. 144). Given the expressions A and B, the binding operation produces a new expression (A, B →{A,B}). A separate procedure then *labels* the output. This work is encouraging in one important respect. Traditionally, a major obstacle to collaboration between neuroscientists and linguists was the abstruseness and intractability of transformational-generative rules. Simplification of these rules at least makes interdisciplinary collaboration possible and should be seen as a step in the right direction, inasmuch as many linguists now seem to have an eye to fundamental neural computations.

Returning to reuse, as I suggested, the most straightforward outcome on the table is for the higher-level ontology to incorporate the lower-level one—i.e., the level of fundamental computations performed in modules and discrete brain regions. But what is the nature of these primitives? Are we talking about discrete domain-general computations in specific cortical sites, with a one-to-one mapping between primitives and brain regions (in the manner contended by Russell Poldrack)? Or are we talking more about dispositions, so that an individual brain region represents a particular complex of primitives, with a many-to-many mapping between primitives and brain regions (in the manner contended by Michael Anderson)? Then there is the issue of how faculty psychology is to proceed in light of nondecomposition and network dynamics (see my discussion in § 5.1). Some structures (maybe many?), as we saw, are not classically decomposable—their properties are not additive in a bottom-up sort of fashion—even though functional decomposition is virtually an article of faith in cognitive science. These are questions to be clarified and hopefully resolved in coming years. What they provide is a sense of the terms that any negotiated settlement between psychology and neuroscience is likely to take, since it is certain that faculty psychology will have to reckon with these primitives one way or another.

8.4 Summary

Multiple realization should not be taken as an empirical given—establishing that a kind is multiply realizable takes a good deal of work, as Shapiro has been at pains to show; and even when the existence of an MR kind can be verified, the details of its implementation do not suddenly become irrelevant. Structure and function are two sides of the same coin. Thus the multiple realization argument provides no basis for neglecting the discoveries of neuroscience. Faculty psychology's strength lies precisely in its willingness to work with neuroscience.

9

Summing Up

This book has been concerned with a specific feature of the organization of biological systems. Livers, hair, eyes, skin, hearts—each exhibits in its own way a certain richness of inner structure it would be foolish to suppose stops the moment one reaches the brain. Happily, no one denies the brain's intricacy of structure and function. The debate has always been over what form this complexity takes. The most influential answer to this question for over 60 years—and the most controversial for almost 40—is that the mind is composed of modules. I took the canonical expression of this concept from Fodor, but isolated it from some of its peculiarities, most especially the notion of strict domain specificity and sensory transduction. I put this refined concept to the test and ended up with a mixed bag of results. Fodorian modules survive in some ways, but die in others. The modules that survive are functionally and anatomically exiguous when set against those postulated by mainstream evolutionary psychologists. They do not handle gross cognitive functions. In effect, they are the columns that Vernon Mountcastle originally hypothesized some 60 years ago, and form part of the well-known "columnar hypothesis" in neuroscience. These modules extend throughout the cortex, so there can be no real sense in which central systems are not modular. This is to say that the cortex appears to be modular in the general sense that it exhibits a limited (and as yet undetermined) degree of functional specialization consistent with the reuse of neural resources. There seems to be no particular difference in this regard between peripheral systems and central systems. Low-level sensory systems appear as reliant on domain-general mechanisms as central ones. Perceptual and linguistic systems do not exhibit the defining characteristics of Fodorian modularity.

Still, the fate of this revised notion of modularity is not certain. The main issue confronting modularity in this revised sense is the effect of neural network context on local function. At some point, the effects of context are so strong that the degree of specialization required for modularity cannot be met. This does not mean that such brain regions are infinitely plastic, prey entirely to the whims of the neural network in which they find themselves: their

The Adaptable Mind. John Zerilli, Oxford University Press (2021). © Oxford University Press.
DOI: 10.1093/oso/9780190067885.003.0009

plasticity is actually impressively constrained, and they exhibit a considerable degree of developmental robustness. Nevertheless, the extent of strong context effects may turn out to be great enough to put a decisive end to modularity's long reign. Recent work in neurobiology is thus forcing a redefinition of the architecture of cognition, principally in terms of patterns of interconnectivity, partial specialization, and emergent specialization. As Giordana Grossi summarizes recent trends:

> . . . cognitive and brain systems that are specialized in adults develop in a highly interconnected brain where regions co-develop with other brain regions, not in isolation. What a brain region or neuron does, in terms of function, depends on its interaction with other regions and neurons[;] it even depends on the state of distributed neural networks. . . . Within this framework, the specialization of neural systems (modularity) assumes a different meaning, one that is anchored into the physical system of a developing organism. . . . (2014, p. 346)

Turning to the language module, we saw that there probably *is* no such thing, not at any rate in the conventional sense, and that dissociations that are otherwise compelling evidence of domain specificity can be adequately explained by the Redundancy Model, which predicates functional inheritance across tasks and task categories even when the tasks are implemented in spatially segregated neural networks.

All up, this is a brave new world. It offers a clearer, cleaner, and far more realistic picture of how the mind works. It is respectful of advances in psychology and philosophy over the past half century, but is anchored firmly in the neurobiological evidence. It strikes what I think is an ideal balance between different approaches to the investigation of the mind/brain. I hope it proves as clarifying and useful to others as it has to me.

References

Aizawa, K. (2009). Neuroscience and multiple realization: A reply to Bechtel and Mundale. *Synthese, 167*(3), 493–510.

Altun, Z. F., & Hall, D. H. (2011). Nervous system, general description. In: *WormAtlas*, eds. Z. F. Altun, L. A. Herndon, C. Crocker, R. Lints, & D. H. Hall. Available at: http://www.wormatlas.org/ver1/handbook/contents.htm.

Amaral, D. G., & Strick, P. L. (2013). The organization of the central nervous system. In: *Principles of neural science*, eds. E. R. Kandel, J. H. Schwartz, T. M. Jessell, S. A. Siegelbaum, & A. J. Hudspeth, pp. 337–355. New York: McGraw-Hill.

Anderson, M. L. (2007a). Evolution of cognitive function via redeployment of brain areas. *The Neuroscientist, 13*, 13–21.

Anderson, M. L. (2007b). Massive redeployment, exaptation, and the functional integration of cognitive operations. *Synthese, 159*(3), 329–345.

Anderson, M. L. (2007c). The massive redeployment hypothesis and the functional topography of the brain. *Philosophical Psychology, 21*(2), 143–174.

Anderson, M. L. (2008). Circuit sharing and the implementation of intelligent systems. *Connection Science, 20*(4), 239–251.

Anderson, M. L. (2010). Neural reuse: A fundamental organizational principle of the brain. *Behavioral and Brain Sciences, 33*(4), 245–266; discussion 266–313.

Anderson, M. L. (2014). *After phrenology: Neural reuse and the interactive brain.* Cambridge, MA: MIT Press.

Anderson, M. L. (2015). Mining the brain for a new taxonomy of the mind. *Philosophy Compass, 10*(1), 68–77.

Anderson, M. L., & Finlay, B. L. (2014). Allocating structure to function: The strong links between neuroplasticity and natural selection. *Frontiers in Human Neuroscience, 7*, 1–16.

Apperly, I. A., Samson, D., Carroll, N., Hussain, S., & Humphreys, G. (2006). Intact first- and second-order false belief reasoning in a patient with severely impaired grammar. *Social Neuroscience, 1*(3–4), 334–348.

Arbib, M. A. (1989). Modularity, schemas and neurons: A critique of Fodor. In: *Computers, brains and minds*, eds. P. Slezak & W. R. Albury, pp. 193–219. Dordrecht: Kluwer.

Ariew, A. (1996). Innateness and canalization. *Philosophy of Science, 63*, S19–S27.

Ariew, A. (1999). Innateness is canalization: In defense of a developmental account of innateness. In: *Where biology meets psychology: Philosophical essays*, ed. V. G. Hardcastle, pp. 117–138. Cambridge, MA: MIT Press.

Ariew, A. (2007). Innateness. In: *Handbook of the philosophy of science: Philosophy of biology*, eds. M. Matthen & C. Stephens, pp. 567–584. Dordrecht: Elsevier.

Avital, E., & Jablonka, E. (2000). *Animal traditions: Behavioural inheritance in evolution.* Cambridge: Cambridge University Press.

Bach-y-Rita, P. (2004). Emerging concepts of brain function. *Journal of Integrative Neuroscience, 4*(2), 183–205.

Badcock, P. B., Ploeger, A., & Allen, N. B. (2016). After phrenology: Time for a paradigm shift in cognitive science. *Behavioral and Brain Sciences,39*, 10–11.

Barrett, H. C. (2006). Modularity and design reincarnation. In: *The innate mind, volume 2: Culture and cognition*, eds. P. Carruthers, S. Laurence, & S. P. Stich, pp. 199–217. New York: Oxford University Press.

Barrett, H. C., & Kurzban, R. (2006). Modularity in cognition: Framing the debate. *Psychological Review, 113*(3), 628–647.

Bates, E. (1999). Plasticity, localization, and language development. In: *The changing nervous system: Neurobehavioral consequences of early brain disorders*, eds. S. H. Broman & J. M. Fletcher, pp. 214–253. New York: Oxford University Press.

Bateson, P., & Mameli, M. (2007). The innate and the acquired: Useful clusters or a residual distinction from folk biology? *Developmental Psychobiology, 49*, 818–831.

Bechtel, W. (2008a). Mechanisms in cognitive psychology: What are the operations? *Philosophy of Science, 75*(5), 983–994.

Bechtel, W. (2008b). *Mental mechanisms: Philosophical perspectives on cognitive neuroscience*. London: Routledge.

Bechtel, W., & Mundale, J. (1999). Multiple realizability revisited: Linking cognitive and neural states. *Philosophy of Science, 66*(2), 175–207.

Bergeron, V. (2007). Anatomical and functional modularity in cognitive science: Shifting the focus. *Philosophical Psychology, 20*(2), 175–195.

Bergeron, V. (2008). Cognitive architecture and the brain: Beyond domain-specific functional specification. Unpublished doctoral dissertation, Department of Philosophy, University of British Columbia. Available at: http://circle.ubc.ca/handle/2429/2711.

Berwick, R. C., & Chomsky, N. (2016). *Why only us: Language and evolution*. Cambridge, MA: MIT Press.

Bickle, J. (1998). *Psychoneural reduction: The new wave*. Cambridge, MA: MIT Press.

Bickle, J. (2003). *Philosophy and neuroscience: A ruthlessly reductive account*. Dordrecht: Springer.

Bickle, J. (2010). Has the last decade of challenges to the multiple realization argument provided aid and comfort to psychoneural reductionists? *Synthese, 177*(2), 247–260.

Binkofski, F., Amunts, K., Stephan, K. M., Posse, S., Schormann, T., Freund, H.-J., Zilles, K., & Seitz, R. J. (2000). Broca's region subserves imagery of motion: A combined cyto-architectonic and fMRI study. *Human Brain Mapping, 11*, 273–285.

Bloom, P. (2000). *How children learn the meanings of words*. Cambridge, MA: MIT Press.

Boone, W., & Piccinini, G. (2016). The cognitive neuroscience revolution. *Synthese,193*, 1509–1534.

Boyd, R., Richerson, P. J., & Henrich, J. (2011). The cultural niche: Why social learning is essential for human adaptation. *Proceedings of the National Academy of Sciences of the United States of America, 108*(Supplement 2), 10918–10925.

Brattico, P., & Liikkanen, L. (2009). Rethinking the Cartesian theory of linguistic productivity. *Philosophical Psychology, 22*(3), 251–279.

Bregman, A. S., & Pinker, S. (1978). Auditory streaming and the building of timbre. *Canadian Journal of Psychology,32*(1), 19–31.

Bressler, S. L. (1995). Large-scale cortical networks and cognition. *Brain Research Reviews, 20*, 288–304.

Bridgeman, B. (2010). Neural reuse implies distributed coding. *Behavioral and Brain Sciences, 33*(4), 269–270.

Brighton, H., Kirby, S., & Smith, K. (2005). Cultural selection for learnability: Three principles underlying the view that language adapts to be learnable. In: *Language origins: Perspectives on evolution*, ed. M. Tallerman, pp. 291–309. Oxford: Oxford University Press.

Bullmore, E., & Sporns, O. (2012). The economy of brain network organization. *Nature Reviews Neuroscience, 13*(5), 336–349.

Buonomano, D. V., & Merzenich, M. M. (1998). Cortical plasticity: From synapses to maps. *Annual Review of Neuroscience, 21*, 149–186.

Burnston, D. C. (2016). A contextualist approach to functional localization in the brain. *Biology and Philosophy, 31*, 527–550.

Buxhoeveden, D. P., & Casanova, M. F. (2002). The minicolumn hypothesis in neuroscience. *Brain, 125*, 935–951.

Cain, D. P. (2001). Synaptic models of neuroplasticity: What is LTP? In: *Toward a theory of neuroplasticity*, eds. C. A. Shaw & J. C. McEachern, pp. 118–129. Philadelphia: Psychology Press.

Caldarelli, G., & Catanzaro, M. (2012). *Networks: A very short introduction.* Oxford: Oxford University Press.

Carandini, M. (2015). From circuits to behavior: A bridge too far? In: *The future of the brain*, eds. G. Marcus & J. Freeman, pp. 177–185. Princeton: Princeton University Press.

Carruthers, P. (2006). *The architecture of the mind: Massive modularity and the flexibility of thought*. Oxford: Oxford University Press.

Carruthers, P. (2008). Précis of *The architecture of the mind: Massive modularity and the flexibility of thought. Mind and Language*, 23(3), 257–262.

Casasanto, D., & Dijkstra, K. (2010). Motor action and emotional memory. *Cognition, 115*(1), 179–185.

Chao, L. L., & Martin, A. (2000). Representation of manipulable man-made objects in the dorsal stream. *NeuroImage, 12*, 478–484.

Chomsky, N. (1956). Three models for the description of language. *IRE transactions on information theory* IT-2: 113–124. Reprinted, with corrections, in: *Readings in mathematical psychology*, Vol. II, eds. R. D. Luce, R. R. Bush, & E. Gallanter, pp. 105–124. New York: John Wiley, & Sons, 1965. References are to the reprint.

Chomsky, N. (1957). *Syntactic structures*. Berlin: Mouton de Gruyter.

Chomsky, N. (1965). *Aspects of the theory of syntax*. Cambridge, MA: MIT Press.

Chomsky, N. (1975). *Reflections on language*. New York: Pantheon.

Chomsky, N. (1979). *Language and responsibility* (with Mitsou Ronat). New York: Pantheon.

Chomsky, N. (1980a). *Rules and representations*. New York: Columbia University Press.

Chomsky, N. (1980b). Rules and representations. *Behavioral and Brain Sciences, 3*(1), 1–15; discussion 15–61.

Chomsky, N. (1988). *Language and problems of knowledge: The Managua lectures*. Cambridge, MA: MIT Press.

Chomsky, N. (1995). *The minimalist program*. Cambridge, MA: MIT Press.

Chomsky, N. (2002). *On nature and language*. New York: Cambridge University Press.

Chomsky, N. (2005). Three factors in language design. *Linguistic Inquiry, 36*(1), 1–22.

Chomsky, N. (2006). *Language and mind*. 3rd ed. New York: Cambridge University Press.

Chomsky, N. (2010). Some simple evo devo theses: How true might they be for language? In: *The evolution of human language: Biolinguistic perspectives*, eds. R. K. Larson, V. Déprez, & H. Yamakido, pp. 45–72. New York: Cambridge University Press.

Chomsky, N. (2016). Minimal computation and the architecture of language. *Chinese Semiotic Studies, 12*(1), 13–24.

Chomsky, N. (2018). Two notions of modularity. In: *On concepts, modules, and language: Cognitive science at its core*, eds. R. G. de Almeida & L. R. Gleitman, pp. 25–40. New York: Oxford University Press.

Christiansen, M. H., & Chater, N. (2016). *Creating language: Integrating evolution, acquisition, and processing.* Cambridge, MA: MIT Press.

Clark, A. (2013). Whatever next? Predictive brains, situated agents, and the future of cognitive science. *Behavioral and Brain Sciences, 36*(3), 181–204; discussion 204–253.

Clark, E. (2009). *First language acquisition.* 2nd ed. Cambridge: Cambridge University Press.

Coase, R. H. (1937). The nature of the firm. *Economica New Series, 4*(16), 386–405.

Cohen, L.G, Celnik, P., Pascual-Leone, A., Corwell, B., Faiz, L., Dambrosia, J., Honda, M., Sadato, N., Gerloff, C., Catalá, M. D., & Hallett, M. (1997). Functional relevance of cross-modal plasticity in blind humans. *Nature, 389*(6647), 180–183.

Cole, M. W., Reynolds, J. R., Power, J. D., Repovs, G., Anticevic, A., & Braver, T. S. (2013). Multi-task connectivity reveals flexible hubs for adaptive task control. *Nature Neuroscience, 16*(9), 1348–1355.

Collins, J. (2004). Faculty disputes. *Mind and Language, 19*(5), 503–533.

Collins, J. (2005). Nativism: In defense of a biological understanding. *Philosophical Psychology, 18*(2), 157–177.

Collins, J. (2008). *Chomsky: A guide for the perplexed.* London: Continuum.

Collins, J. (2004). Brain imaging, connectionism, and cognitive neuropsychology. *Cognitive Neuropsychology, 21*(1), 21–25.

Collins, J. (2011). Methods for modular modelling: Additive factors and cognitive neuropsychology. *Cognitive Neuropsychology, 28*(3–4), 224–240.

Coltheart, M. (1999). Modularity and cognition. *Trends in Cognitive Sciences, 3*(3), 115–120.

Cosmides, L., & Tooby, J. (1994). Origins of domain specificity: The evolution of functional organization. In: *Mapping the world: Domain specificity in cognition and culture*, eds. L. Hirschfield & S. Gelman, pp. 85–116. New York: Cambridge University Press.

Couch, M. B. (2009). Functional explanation in context. *Philosophy of Science, 76*(2), 253–269.

Cowie, F. (2008). Innateness and language. In: *The Stanford encyclopedia of philosophy*, winter 2016, ed. E. N. Zalta. Available at: http://plato.stanford.edu/archives/win2016/entries/innateness-language/.

Craver, C. F. (2007). *Explaining the brain.* Oxford: Oxford University Press.

Croft, W., & Cruise, D. A. (2004). *Cognitive linguistics.* Cambridge: Cambridge University Press.

da Costa, N. M., & Martin, K. A. C. (2010). Whose cortical column would that be? *Frontiers in Neuroanatomy, 4*(5), 1–10.

Damasio, A. R., & Tranel, D. (1993). Nouns and verbs are retrieved with differently distributed neural systems. *Proceedings of the National Academy of Sciences of the United States of America, 90*, 4957–4960.

Damasio, H., Grabowski, T. J., Tranel, D., Hichwa, R. D., & Damasio, A. R. (1996). A neural basis for lexical retrieval. *Science, 380*, 499–505.

Danelli, L., Cossu, G., Berlingeri, M., Bottini, G., Sberna, M., & Paulesu, E. (2013). Is a lone right hemisphere enough? Neurolinguistic architecture in a case with a very early left hemispherectomy. *Neurocase,19*(3), 209–231.

de Boer, B. (2016). Evolution of speech and evolution of language. *Psychonomic Bulletin and Review,* 2016, 1–5. doi: 10.3758/s13423-016-1130-6.

Deacon, T. W. (1997). *The symbolic species: The co-evolution of language and the brain.* New York: Norton.

Deacon, T. W. (2010). A role for relaxed selection in the evolution of the language capacity. *Proceedings of the National Academy of Sciences of the United States of America, 107,* 9000–9006.

Decety, J., Grèzes, J., Costes, N., Perani, D., Jeannerod, M., Procyk, E., Grassi, F., & Fazio, F. (1997). Brain activity during observation of actions. Influence of action content and subject's strategy. *Brain, 120*(10), 1763–1777.

Dehaene, S. (2005). Evolution of human cortical circuits for reading and arithmetic: The "neuronal recycling" hypothesis. In: *From monkey brain to human brain,* eds. S. Dehaene, J. R. Duhamel, M. D. Hauser, & G. Rizzolatti, pp. 133–157. Cambridge, MA: MIT Press.

Dehaene, S., Bossini, S., & Giraux, P. (1993). The mental representation of parity and numerical magnitude. *Journal of Experimental Psychology: General, 122,* 371–396.

Dennett, D. C. (1991). *Consciousness explained.* London: Penguin.

Doidge, N. (2007). *The brain that changes itself.* New York: Penguin.

Dor, D., & Jablonka, E. (2010). Canalization and plasticity in the evolution of linguistic communication: An evolutionary developmental approach. In: *The evolution of human language: Biolinguistic perspectives,* eds. R. K. Larson, V. Déprez, & H. Yamakido, pp. 135–147. New York: Cambridge University Press.

Dunn, M., Greenhill, S. J., Levinson, S. C., & Gray, R. D. (2011). Evolved structure of language shows lineage-specific trends in word-order universals. *Nature, 473,* 79–82.

Edelman, G. M., & Gally, J. A. (2001). Degeneracy and complexity in biological systems. *Proceedings of the National Academy of Sciences of the United States of America, 98*(24), 13763–13768.

Elbert, T., Pantev, C., Wienbruch, C., Rockstroh, B., & Taub, E. (1995). Increased cortical representation of the fingers of the left hand in string players. *Science, 270,* 305–307.

Eliasmith, C. (2015). Building a behaving brain. In: *The future of the brain,* eds. G. Marcus & J. Freeman, pp. 125–136. Princeton: Princeton University Press.

Evans, N., & Levinson, S. C. (2009). The myth of language universals: Language diversity and its importance for cognitive science. *Behavioral and Brain Sciences, 32*(5), 429–448; discussion 448–492.

Evans, V., & Green, M. (2006). *Cognitive linguistics: An introduction.* Edinburgh: Edinburgh University Press.

Everett, D. (2012). *Language: The cultural tool.* New York: Vintage.

Fedorenko, E., Behr, M. K., & Kanwisher, N. (2011). Functional specificity for high-level linguistic processing in the human brain. *Proceedings of the National Academy of Sciences of the United States of America,108*(39), 16428–16433.

Fedorenko, E., Duncan, J., & Kanwisher, N. (2012). Language-selective and domain-general regions lie side by side within Broca's area. *Current Biology,22*(21), 2059–2062.

Fedorenko, E., & Thompson-Schill, S. L. (2014). Reworking the language network. *Trends in Cognitive Sciences, 18*(3), 120–126.

Fisher, S. E. (2015). Translating the genome in human neuroscience. In: *The future of the brain*, eds. G. Marcus & J. Freeman, pp. 149–158. Princeton: Princeton University Press.

Fisher, S. E., & Scharff, C. (2009). *FOXP2* as a molecular window into speech and language. *Trends in Genetics, 25*, 166–177.

Fitch, W. T. (2010). Three meanings of "recursion": Key distinctions for biolinguistics. In: *The evolution of human language: Biolinguistic perspectives*, eds. R. K. Larson, V. Déprez, & H. Yamakido, pp. 73–90. New York: Cambridge University Press.

Fitch, W. T., Hauser, M. D., & Chomsky, N. (2005). The evolution of the language faculty: Clarifications and implications. *Cognition, 97*, 179–210.

Fodor, J. A. (1975). *The language of thought*. Cambridge, MA: Harvard University Press.

Fodor, J. A. (1983). *The modularity of mind: An essay on faculty psychology*. Cambridge, MA: MIT Press.

Fodor, J. A., Bever, T., & Garrett, M. (1974). *The psychology of language: An introduction to psycholinguistics and generative grammar*. New York: McGraw-Hill.

Frost, R., Armstrong, B. C., Siegelman, N., & Christiansen, M. H. (2015). Domain generality versus modality specificity: The paradox of statistical learning. *Trends in Cognitive Sciences, 19*(3), 117–125.

Fuchs, E., & Flügge, G. (2014). Adult neuroplasticity: More than 40 years of research. *Neural Plasticity, 2014*, 1–10. doi: 10.1155/2014/541870.

Gall, F. J., & Spurzheim, J. C. (1835). *On the function of the brain and each of its parts*. Boston: Marsh Capen and Lyon.

Gauthier, I., Curran, T., Curby, K. M., & Collins, D. (2003). Perceptual interference supports a non-modular account of face processing. *Nature Neuroscience, 6*(4), 428–432.

Gauthier, I., Skudlarski, P. Gore, J. C., & Anderson, A. W. (2000). Expertise for cars and birds recruits brain areas involved in face recognition. *Nature Neuroscience, 3*(2), 191–197.

Gazzaniga, M. S. (1989). Organization of the human brain. *Science, 245*(4921), 947–952.

Gerrans, P. (2014). *The measure of madness: Philosophy of mind, cognitive neuroscience, and delusional thought*. Cambridge, MA: MIT Press.

Gilbert, C. D. (2013). The constructive nature of visual processing. In: *Principles of neural science*, eds. E. R. Kandel, J. H. Schwartz, T. M. Jessell, S. A. Siegelbaum, & A. J. Hudspeth, pp. 556–576. New York: McGraw-Hill.

Gillett, C. (2002). The dimensions of realization: A critique of the standard view. *Analysis, 62*(4), 316–323.

Gillett, C. (2003). The metaphysics of realization, multiple realizability, and the special sciences. *Journal of Philosophy, 100*(11), 591–603.

Glenberg, A. M., Brown, M., & Levin, J. R. (2007). Enhancing comprehension in small reading groups using a manipulation strategy. *Contemporary Educational Psychology, 32*, 389–399.

Glenberg, A. M., Sato, M., & Cattaneo, L. (2008). Use-induced motor plasticity affects the processing of abstract and concrete language. *Current Biology, 18*(7), R290–R291.

Glickstein, M. (2014). *Neuroscience: A historical introduction*. Cambridge, MA: MIT Press.

Godfrey-Smith, P. (2001). Three kinds of adaptationism. In: *Adaptationism and optimality*, ed. S. H. Orzack & E. Sober, pp. 335–357. Cambridge: Cambridge University Press.

Gold, I., & Roskies, A. L. (2008). Philosophy of neuroscience. In: *The Oxford handbook of philosophy of biology*, ed. M. Ruse, pp. 349–380. New York: Oxford University Press.

Goldberg, A. E. (2003). Constructions: A new theoretical approach to language. *Trends in Cognitive Sciences, 7*(5), 219–224.

Graziano, M. S. A., Taylor, C. S. R., Moore, T., & Cooke, D. F. (2002). The cortical control of movement revisited. *Neuron, 36,* 349–362.

Greenfield, P. M. (1991). Language, tools and brain: The ontogeny and phylogeny of hierarchically organized sequential behavior. *Behavioral and Brain Sciences, 14*(4), 531–551; discussion 551–595.

Greenhill, S. J., Atkinson, Q. D., Meade, A., & Gray, R. D. (2010). The shape and tempo of language evolution. *Proceedings of the Royal Society B: Biological Sciences, 277,* 2443–2450.

Griffiths, P. E. (2002). What is innateness? *Monist, 85,* 70–85.

Griffiths, P. E., & Machery, E. (2008). Innateness, canalization, and "biologicizing the mind." *Philosophical Psychology, 21*(3), 397–414.

Griffiths, P. E., Machery, E., & Linquist, S. (2009). The vernacular concept of innateness. *Mind and Language, 24*(5), 605–630.

Grossi, G. (2014). A module is a module is a module: Evolution of modularity in evolutionary psychology. *Dialectical Anthropology, 38,* 333–351.

Gruber, O. (2002). The co-evolution of language and working memory capacity in the human brain. In: *Mirror neurons and the evolution of brain and language,* eds. M. I. Stamenov & V. Gallese, pp. 77–86. Amsterdam: John Benjamins.

Guida, A., Campitelli, G., & Gobet, F. (2016). Becoming an expert: Ontogeny of expertise as an example of neural reuse. *Behavioral and Brain Sciences, 39,* 13–15.

Hagoort, P., & Indefrey, P. (2014). The neurobiology of language beyond single words. *Annual Review of Neuroscience, 37,* 347–362.

Hanson, S. J., Matsuka, T., & Haxby, J. V. (2004). Combinatorial codes in ventral temporal lobe for object recognition: Is there a "face" area? *NeuroImage, 23*(1), 156–166.

Hardcastle, V. G., & Stewart, C. M. (2009). fMRI: A modern cerebrascope? The case of pain. In: *The Oxford handbook of philosophy and neuroscience,* ed. J. Bickle, pp. 179–199. New York: Oxford University Press.

Hauser, M. D., Chomsky, N., & Fitch, W. T. (2002). The faculty of language: What is it, who has it and how did it evolve? *Science, 298*(5598), 1569–1579.

Hawrylycz, M. (2015). Building atlases of the brain. In: *The future of the brain,* eds. G. Marcus & J. Freeman, pp. 3–16. Princeton: Princeton University Press.

Haxby, J. V., Gobbini, M. I., Furey, M. L., Ishai, A., Schouten, J. L., & Pietrini, P. (2001). Distributed and overlapping representations of faces and objects in ventral temporal cortex. *Science, 293,* 2425–2430.

Hebb, D. O. (1949). *The organization of behavior: A neuropsychological theory.* New York: Wiley.

Hickok, G., & Poeppel, D. (2000). Towards a functional neuroanatomy of speech perception. *Trends in Cognitive Sciences, 4*(4), 131–138.

Hirst, P., Khomami, P. J., Gharat, A., & Zangenehpour, S. (2012). Cross-modal recruitment of primary visual cortex by auditory stimuli in the nonhuman primate brain: A molecular mapping study. *Neural Plasticity, 2012,* 1–11. doi: 10.1155/2012/197264.

Horst, S. W. (2011). *Laws, mind, and free will.* Cambridge, MA: MIT Press.

Hsu, H. J., Tomblin, J. B., & Christiansen, M. H. (2014). Impaired statistical learning of non-adjacent dependencies in adolescents with specific language impairment. *Frontiers in Psychology, 5,* 175.

Hubbard, E. M., Piazza, M., Pinel, P., & Dehaene, S. (2005). Interactions between number and space in parietal cortex. *Nature Reviews Neuroscience, 6*(6), 435–448.

Iriki, A., & Taoka, M. (2012). Triadic (ecological, neural, cognitive) niche construction: A scenario of human brain evolution extrapolating tool use and language from the control of reaching actions. *Philosophical Transactions of the Royal Society B, 367,* 10–23.

Jackendoff, R. (2007). A Parallel Architecture perspective on language processing. *Brain Research, 1146,* 2–22.

Jacobs, J. A. (1999). Computational studies of the development of functionally specialized neural modules. *Trends in Cognitive Sciences,3*(1), 31–38.

Jilk, D. J., Lebiere, C., O'Reilly, R. C., & Anderson, J. R. (2008). SAL: An explicitly pluralistic cognitive architecture. *Journal of Experimental and Theoretical Artificial Intelligence, 20,* 197–218.

Jungé, J. A., & Dennett, D. C. (2010). Multi-use and constraints from original use. *Behavioral and Brain Sciences, 33*(4), 277–278.

Jusczyk, P. W., & Cohen, A. (1985). What constitutes a module? *Behavioral and Brain Sciences, 8*(1), 20–21.

Kaan, E., & Stowe, L. A. (2002). Storage and computation in the brain: A neuroimaging perspective. In: *Storage and computation in the language faculty*, eds. S. G. Nooteboom, F. Weerman, & F. N. K. Wijnen, pp. 257–298. Dordrecht: Kluwer.

Kaan, E., & Swaab, T. Y. (2002). The brain circuitry of syntactic comprehension. *Trends in Cognitive Sciences, 6*(8), 350–356.

Kandel, E. R., Barres, B. A., & Hudspeth, A. J. (2013). Nerve cells, neural circuitry, and behavior. In: *Principles of neural science*, eds. E. R. Kandel, J. H. Schwartz, T. M. Jessell, S. A. Siegelbaum, & A. J. Hudspeth, pp. 21–38. New York: McGraw-Hill.

Kandel, E. R., & Hudspeth, A. J. (2013). The brain and behavior. In: *Principles of neural science*, eds. E. R. Kandel, J. H. Schwartz, T. M. Jessell, S. A. Siegelbaum, & A. J. Hudspeth, pp. 5–20. New York: McGraw-Hill.

Kanwisher, N., McDermott, J., & Chun, M. (1997). The fusiform face area: A module in human extrastriate cortex specialized for face perception. *Journal of Neuroscience, 17*(11), 4302–4311.

Karmiloff-Smith, A. (1992). *Beyond modularity: A developmental perspective on cognitive science.* Cambridge, MA: MIT Press.

Karmiloff-Smith, A. (1994). Précis of *Beyond modularity: A developmental perspective on cognitive science. Behavioral and Brain Sciences, 17*(4), 693–706; discussion 707–745.

Kim, J. (1992). Multiple realization and the metaphysics of reduction. *Philosophy and Phenomenological Research,52*(1), 1–26.

Kim, S. (2002). Testing multiple realizability: A discussion of Bechtel and Mundale. *Philosophy of Science, 69*(4), 606–610.

Kirby, S., Dowman, M., & Griffiths, T. L. (2007). Innateness and culture in the evolution of language. *Proceedings of the National Academy of Sciences of the United States of America, 104,* 5241–5245.

Klein, C. (2008). An ideal solution to disputes about multiply realized kinds. *Philosophical Studies, 140*(2), 161–177.

Klein, C. (2010). Redeployed functions versus spreading activation: A potential confound. *Behavioral and Brain Sciences, 33*(4), 280–281.

Klein, C. (2012). Cognitive ontology and region- versus network-oriented analyses. *Philosophy of Science, 79*(5), 952–960.

Knott, A. (2012*). Sensorimotor cognition and natural language syntax*. Cambridge, MA: MIT Press.

Koch, C. (2015). Project *MindScope*. In: *The future of the brain*, eds. G. Marcus & J. Freeman, pp. 25–39. Princeton: Princeton University Press.

Kolb, B., Gibb. R., & Gonzalez, C. L. R. (2001). Cortical injury and neuroplasticity during brain development. In: *Toward a theory of neuroplasticity*, eds. C. A. Shaw & J. C. McEachern, pp. 223–243. Philadelphia: Psychology Press.

Krubitzer, L. (1995). The organization of neocortex in mammals: Are species differences really so different? *Trends in Neurosciences, 18*(9), 408–417.

Kuhl, P. K., & Damasio, A. R. (2013). Language. In: *Principles of neural science*, eds. E. R. Kandel, J. H. Schwartz, T. M. Jessell, S. A. Siegelbaum, & A. J. Hudspeth, pp. 1353–1372. New York: McGraw-Hill.

Lai, C. S. L., Fisher, S. E., Hurst, J. A., Vargha-Khadem, F., & Monaco, A. P. (2001). A forkhead-domain gene is mutated in a severe speech and language disorder. *Nature, 413*, 519–523.

Laland, K. N. (2016). The origins of language in teaching. *Psychonomic Bulletin and Review*, 2016, 1–7. doi: 10.3758/s13423-016-1077-7.

Laland, K. N. Sterelny, K., Odling-Smee, J., Hoppit, W., & Uller, T. (2011). Cause and effect in biology revisited: Is Mayr's proximate-ultimate dichotomy still useful? *Science, 334*(6062), 1512–1516.

Laland, K.N, Uller, T., Feldman, M. W., Sterelny, K., Müller, G. B., Moczek, A., Jablonka, E., & Odling-Smee, J. (2015). The extended evolutionary synthesis: Its structure, assumptions and predictions. *Proceedings of the Royal Society B, 282*, 20151019.

Landon, B. (2013). *Building great sentences: How to write the kinds of sentences you love to read*. Penguin: New York.

Laurence, S., & Margolis, E. (2015). Concept nativism and neural plasticity. In: *The conceptual mind: New directions in the study of concepts*, eds. E. Margolis & S. Laurence, pp. 117–147. Cambridge, MIT: MIT Press.

Leiber, J. (2006). Turing's golden: How well Turing's work stands today. *Philosophical Psychology, 19*(1), 13–46.

Leise, E. M. (1990). Modular construction of nervous systems: A basic principle of design for invertebrates and vertebrates. *Brain Research Reviews, 15*, 1–23.

Leo, A., Bernardi, G., Handjaras, G., Bonino, D., Ricciardi, E., & Pietrini, P. (2012). Increased BOLD variability in the parietal cortex and enhanced parieto-occipital connectivity during tactile perception in congenitally blind individuals. *Neural Plasticity*, 2012, 1–8. doi: 10.1155/2012/720278.

Levinson, S. C. (2000). *Presumptive meanings: The theory of generalized conversational implicature*. Cambridge, MA: MIT Press.

Lingnau, A., Strnad, L., He, C., Fabbri, S., Han, Z., Bi, Y., & Caramazza, A. (2014). Cross-modal plasticity preserves functional specialization in posterior parietal cortex. *Cerebral Cortex, 24*, 541–549.

Liu, L., & Kager, R. (2016). Enhanced music sensitivity in 9-month-old bilingual infants. *Cognitive Processing*, 2016, 1–11. doi: 10.1007/s10339-016-0780-7.

Luria, A. R., Tsvetkova, L. S., & Futer, D. S. (1965). Aphasia in a composer (V. G. Shebalin). *Journal of the Neurological Sciences, 2*(3), 288–292.

MacDermot, K. D., Bonora, E., Sykes, N. Coupe, A. M., Lai, C. S. L., Vernes, S. C., Vargha-Khadem, F., McKenzie, F., Smith, R. L., Monaco, A. P., & Fisher, S. E. (2005).

Identification of *FOXP2* truncation as a novel cause of developmental speech and language deficits. *American Journal of Human Genetics, 76*(6), 1074–1080.

MacNeilage, P. F. (1998). The frame/content theory of evolution of speech production. *Behavioral and Brain Sciences,21*(4), 499–511; discussion 511–546.

Maess, B., Koelsch, S., Gunter, T. C., & Friederici, A. D. (2001). Musical syntax is processed in Broca's area: An MEG study. *Nature Neuroscience, 4*, 540–545.

Mahon, B. Z., & Cantlon, J. F. (2011). The specialization of function: Cognitive and neural perspectives. *Cognitive Neuropsychology, 28*(3–4), 147–155.

Maleszka, R., Mason, P. H., & Barron, A. B. (2013). Epigenomics and the concept of degeneracy in biological systems. *Briefings in Functional Genomics, 13*(3), 191–202.

Malle, B. F. (2002). The relation between language and theory of mind in development and evolution. In: *The evolution of language out of pre-language*, eds. T. Givón & B. Malle, pp. 265–284. Philadelphia: John Benjamins.

Mameli, M., & Bateson, P. (2006). Innateness and the sciences. *Biology and Philosophy, 21*, 155–188.

Mameli, M., & Bateson, P. (2011). An evaluation of the concept of innateness. *Philosophical Transactions of the Royal Society B, 366*, 436–443.

Mameli, M., & Papineau, D. (2006). The new nativism: A commentary on Gary Marcus's *The birth of the mind. Biology and Philosophy, 21*, 559–573.

Mampe, B., Friederici, A. D., Christophe, A., & Wermke, K. (2009). Newborns' cry melody is shaped by their native language. *Current Biology,19*(23), 1994–1997.

Marcus, G. (2004). *The birth of the mind: How a tiny number of genes creates the complexities of human thought.* New York: Basic Books.

Marr, D. (1976). Early processing of visual information. *Philosophical Transactions of the Royal Society B, 275*, 483–524.

Marr, D. (2010 [1982]). *Vision: A computational investigation into the human representation and processing of visual information.* Cambridge, MA: MIT Press.

Martin, A., Haxby, J. V., Lalonde, F. M., Wiggs, C. L., & Ungerleider, L. G. (1995). Discrete cortical regions associated with knowledge of color and knowledge of action. *Science, 270*, 102–105.

Martin, A., Ungerleider, L. G., & Haxby, J. V. (2000). Category-specificity and the brain: The sensorymotor model of semantic representations of objects. In: *The new cognitive neurosciences*, 2nd ed., ed. M. S. Gazzaniga, pp. 1023–1036. Cambridge, MA, MIT Press.

Martin, A., Wiggs, C. L., Ungerleider, L. G., & Haxby, J. V. (1996). Neural correlates of category-specific knowledge. *Nature, 379*(6566), 649–652.

Mason, P. H. (2010). Degeneracy at multiple levels of complexity. *Biological Theory, 5*(3), 277–288.

Mather, M., Cacioppo, J. T., & Kanwisher, N. (2013). How fMRI can inform cognitive theories. *Perspectives on Psychological Science,8*(1), 108–113.

McGeer, V. (2007). Why neuroscience matters to cognitive neuropsychology. *Synthese, 159*, 347–371.

McGilvray, J. (2014). *Chomsky: Language, mind, politics.* 2nd ed. Cambridge: Polity Press.

Melchner, L., Pallas, S. L., & Sur, M. (2000). Visual behaviour mediated by retinal projections directed to the auditory pathway. *Nature,404*(6780), 871–876.

Merabet, L. B., & Pascual-Leone, A. (2010). Neural organization following sensory loss: The opportunity of change. *Nature Reviews Neuroscience, 11*, 44–52.

Mnih, V., Kavukcuoglu, K., Silver, D., Rusu, A. A., Veness, J., Bellemare, M. G., Graves, A., Riedmiller, M., Fidjeland, A. K., Ostrovski, G., Petersen, S., Beattie, C., Sadik, A., Antonoglou, I., King, H., Kumaran, D., Wierstra, D., Legg, S., & Hassabis, D. (2015). Human-level control through deep reinforcement learning. *Nature, 518,* 529–533.

Moore, R. (2017). The evolution of syntactic structure. *Biology and Philosophy, 32*(4), 599–613.

Mountcastle, V. B. (1957). Modality and topographic properties of single neurons of cat's somatic sensory cortex. *Journal of Neurophysiology, 20*(4), 408–434.

Mountcastle, V. B. (1978). An organizing principle for cerebral function: The unit module and the distributed system. In: *The mindful brain*, eds. G. Edelman & V. B. Mountcastle, pp. 7–50. Cambridge, MA: MIT Press.

Mountcastle, V. B. (1997). The columnar organization of the neocortex. *Brain, 120,* 701–722.

Müller, R.-A., & Basho, S. (2004). Are nonlinguistic functions in "Broca's area" prerequisites for language acquisition? fMRI findings from an ontogenetic viewpoint. *Brain and Language, 89*(2), 329–336.

Neville, H. J., & Bavelier, D. (2001). Specificity of developmental neuroplasticity in humans: Evidence from sensory deprivation and altered language experience. In: *Toward a theory of neuroplasticity*, eds. C. A. Shaw & J. C. McEachern, pp. 261–274. Philadelphia: Psychology Press.

Nishitani, N., Schürmann, M., Amunts, K., & Hari, R. (2005). Broca's region: From action to language. *Physiology, 20,* 60–69.

Noppeney, U. (2007). The effects of visual deprivation on structural and functional organization of the human brain. *Neuroscience and Biobehavioral Reviews, 31,* 1169–1180.

Ohlsson, S. (1994). Representational change, generality versus specificity, and nature versus nurture: Perennial issues in cognitive research. *Behavioral and Brain Sciences, 17*(4), 724–725.

O'Neill, E. (2015). Relativizing innateness: Innateness as the insensitivity of the appearance of a trait with respect to specified environmental variation. *Biology and Philosophy,30,* 211–225.

O'Reilly, R. C. (1998). Six principles for biologically-based computational models of cortical cognition. *Trends in Cognitive Sciences,2*(11), 455–462.

O'Reilly, R. C., Munakata, Y., Frank, M. J., Hazy, T. E., & Contributors. (2012). *Computational cognitive neuroscience.* 1st ed. Wiki Book. Available at: http://ccnbook. colorado.edu.

Parfit, D. (1984). *Reasons and persons.* Oxford: Oxford University Press.

Pascual-Leone, A., Amedi, A., Fregni, F., & Merabet, L. B. (2005). The plastic human brain cortex. *Annual Review of Neuroscience, 28,* 377–401.

Pascual-Leone, A., & Hamilton, R. (2001). The metamodal organization of the brain. *Progress in Brain Research, 134,* 427–445.

Pascual-Leone, A., & Torres, F. (1993). Plasticity of the sensorimotor cortex representation of the reading finger in Braille readers. *Brain, 116,* 39–52.

Pasqualotto, A. (2016). Multisensory integration substantiates distributed and overlapping neural networks. *Behavioral and Brain Sciences, 39,* 20–21.

Peretz, I., & Coltheart, M. (2003). Modularity of music processing. *Nature Neuroscience, 6,* 688–691.

Pessoa, L. (2016). Beyond disjoint brain networks: Overlapping networks for cognition and emotion. *Behavioral and Brain Sciences, 39,* 22–24.

Petrov, A. A., Jilk, D. J., & O'Reilly, R. C. (2010). The Leabra architecture: Specialization without modularity. *Behavioral and Brain Sciences, 33*(4), 286–287.

Piccinini, G., & Craver, C. (2011). Integrating psychology and neuroscience: Functional analyses as mechanism sketches. *Synthese,183*, 283–311.

Pinker, S. (1994). *The language instinct*. London: Penguin/Folio.

Pinker, S. (1997). *How the mind works*. New York: Norton.

Pinker, S., & Jackendoff, R. (2005). The faculty of language: What's special about it? *Cognition, 95*, 201–236.

Plaut, D. C. (1995). Double dissociation without modularity: Evidence from connectionist neuropsychology. *Journal of Clinical and Experimental Psychology,17*(2), 291–321.

Poeppel, D. (2001). Pure word deafness and the bilateral processing of the speech code. *Cognitive Science, 21*(5), 679–693.

Poeppel, D. (2015). The neurobiology of language. In: *The future of the brain*, eds. G. Marcus & J. Freeman, pp. 139–148. Princeton: Princeton University Press.

Poldrack, R. A. (2010). Mapping mental function to brain structure: How can cognitive neuroimaging succeed? *Perspectives on Psychological Science, 5*(6), 753–761.

Poldrack, R. A., Halchenko, Y. O., & Hanson, S. J. (2009). Decoding the large-scale structure of brain function by classifying mental states across individuals. *Psychological Science, 20*(11), 1364–1372.

Polger, T. W. (2008). Two confusions concerning multiple realization. *Philosophy of Science, 75*(5), 537–547.

Polger, T. W. (2009). Evaluating the evidence for multiple realization. *Synthese, 167*(3), 457–472.

Polger, T. W., & Shapiro, L. A. (2008). Understanding the dimensions of realization. *Journal of Philosophy, 105*(4), 213–222.

Polger, T. W., & Shapiro, L. A. (2016). *The multiple realization book*. Oxford: Oxford University Press.

Price, C. J., & Friston, K. J. (2005). Functional ontologies for cognition: The systematic definition of structure and function. *Cognitive Neuropsychology, 22*(3), 262–275.

Prinz, J. J. (2006). Is the mind really modular? In: *Contemporary debates in cognitive science*, ed. R. Stainton, pp. 22–36. Oxford: Blackwell.

Ptito, M., Kupers, R., Lomber, S., & Pietrini, P. (2012). Sensory deprivation and brain plasticity. *Neural Plasticity,* 2012, 1–2. doi: 10.1155/2012/810370.

Ptito, M., Matteau, I., Zhi Wang, A., Paulson, O. B., Siebner, H. R., & Kupers, R. (2012). Crossmodal recruitment of the ventral visual stream in congenital blindness. *Neural Plasticity,* 2012, 1–9. doi: 10.1155/2012/304045.

Pullum, G. K., & Scholz, B. C. (2002). Empirical assessment of stimulus poverty arguments. *Linguistic Review,19*, 9–50.

Pulvermüller, F. (2005). Brain mechanisms linking language and action. *Nature Reviews Neuroscience, 6*, 576–582.

Pulvermüller, F., & Fadiga, L. (2010). Active perception: Sensorimotor circuits as a cortical basis for language. *Nature Reviews Neuroscience, 11*, 351–360.

Putnam, H. (1967). Psychological predicates. In: *Art, mind, and religion*, eds. W. Capitan & D. Merrill, pp. 37–48. Pittsburgh: University of Pittsburgh Press.

Quartz, S. R., & Sejnowski, T. J. (1994). Neural evidence for constructivist principles in development. *Behavioral and Brain Sciences, 17*(4), 725–726.

Ramus, F., & Fisher, S. E. (2009). Genetics of Language. In: *The cognitive neurosciences*, 4th ed., ed. M. S. Gazzaniga, pp. 855–872. Cambridge, MA: MIT Press.

Rasmussen, J. (1986). *Information processing and human-machine interaction.* Amsterdam: North-Holland.

Rauschecker, J. P. (2001). Developmental neuroplasticity within and across sensory modalities. In: *Toward a theory of neuroplasticity*, eds. C. A. Shaw & J. C. McEachern, pp. 244–260. Philadelphia: Psychology Press.

Renier, L. A., Anurova, I., De Volder, A. G., Carlson, S., VanMeter, J., & Rauschecker, J. P. (2010). Preserved functional specialization for spatial processing in the middle occipital gyrus of the early blind. *Neuron, 68*(1), 138–148.

Richerson, P. J., & Boyd, R. (2005). *Not by genes alone: How culture transformed human evolution.* Chicago: University of Chicago Press.

Ritchie, J. B., & Carruthers, P. (2010). Massive modularity is consistent with most forms of neural reuse. *Behavioral and Brain Sciences, 33*(4), 289–290.

Robbins, P. (2009). Modularity of mind. In: *The Stanford encyclopedia of philosophy*, summer 2010, ed. E. N. Zalta. Available at: http://plato.stanford.edu/archives/sum2010/entries/modularity-mind/.

Rockland, K. S. (2010). Five points on columns. *Frontiers in Neuroanatomy, 4*(6), 1–10.

Rose, J. K., & Rankin, C. H. (2001). Behavioral, neural circuit and genetic analyses of habituation in *C. elegans*. In: *Toward a theory of neuroplasticity*, eds. C. A. Shaw & J. C. McEachern, pp. 176–192. Philadelphia: Psychology Press.

Rowland, D. C., & Moser, M. B. (2014). From cortical modules to memories. *Current Opinion in Neurobiology, 24*, 22–27.

Sadato, N., Pascual-Leone, A., Grafman, J., Ibañez, V., Deiber, M. P., Dold, G., & Hallett, M. (1996). Activation of the primary visual cortex by Braille reading in blind subjects. *Nature, 380*(6574), 526–528.

Saitoe, M., & Tully, T. (2001). Making connections between developmental and behavioral plasticity in *Drosophila*. In: *Toward a theory of neuroplasticity*, eds. C. A. Shaw & J. C. McEachern, pp. 193–220. Philadelphia: Psychology Press.

Sanes, J. R., & Jessell, T. M. (2013). Experience and the refinement of synaptic connections. In: *Principles of neural science*, eds. E. R. Kandel, J. H. Schwartz, T. M. Jessell, S. A. Siegelbaum, & A. J. Hudspeth, pp. 1259–1283. New York: McGraw-Hill.

Scholl, B. J. (1997). Neural constraints on cognitive modularity? *Behavioral and Brain Sciences,20*(4), 575–576.

Scholz, B. C., & Pullum, G. K. (2002). Searching for arguments to support linguistic nativism. *Linguistic Review,19*, 185–223.

Schreiweis, C., Bornschein, U., Burguière, E., Kerimoglu, C., Schreiter, S., Dannemann, M., Goyal, S., Rea, E., French, C. A., Puliyadi, R., Groszer, M., Fisher, S. E., Mundry, R., Winter, C., Hevers, W., Pääbo, S., Enard, W., & Graybiel, A. M. (2014). Humanized Foxp2 accelerates learning by enhancing transitions from declarative to procedural performance. *Proceedings of the National Academy of Sciences of the United States of America,111*(39), 14253–14258.

Shapiro, L. A. (2000). Multiple realizations. *Journal of Philosophy, 97*(12), 635–654.

Shapiro, L. A. (2004). *The mind incarnate.* Cambridge, MA: MIT Press.

Shapiro, L. A. (2008). How to test for multiple realization. *Philosophy of Science, 75*(5), 514–525.

Shapiro, L. A., & Polger, T. W. (2012). Identity, variability, and multiple realization in the special sciences. In: *New perspectives on type identity: The mental and the physical*, eds. S. Gozzano & C. S. Hill, pp. 264–286. Cambridge: Cambridge University Press.

Shaw, C. A., & McEachern, J. C., eds. (2001). *Toward a theory of neuroplasticity*. Philadelphia: Psychology Press.

Sharma, J., Angelucci, A., & Sur, M. (2000). Induction of visual orientation modules in auditory cortex. *Nature, 404*(6780), 841–847.

Silberstein, M. (2016). The implications of neural reuse for the future of both cognitive neuroscience and folk psychology. *Behavioral and Brain Sciences, 39*, 27–29.

Smit, H. (2014). *The Social Evolution of Human Nature: From Biology to Language*. Cambridge: Cambridge University Press.

Smith, K., & Kirby, S. (2008). Cultural evolution: Implications for understanding the human language faculty and its evolution. *Philosophical Transactions of the Royal Society B, 363*, 3591–3603.

Sorrells, S. F., Paredes, M. F., Cebrian-Silla, A., Sandoval, K., Qi, D., Kelley, K. W., James, D., Mayer, S., Chang, J., Auguste, J. I., Chang, E. F., Gutierrez, A. J., Kriegstein, A. R., Mathern, A. M., Oldham, M. C., Huang, E. J., Garcia-Verdugo, J. M., Yang, Z., & Alvarez-Buylla, A. (2018). Human hippocampal neurogenesis drops sharply in children to undetectable levels in adults. *Nature, 555*, 377–381.

Sperber, D. (1994). The modularity of thought and the epidemiology of representations. In: *Mapping the mind*, eds. L. A. Hirschfield & S. A. Gelman, pp. 39–67. Cambridge: Cambridge University Press.

Sperber, D. (2002). In defense of massive modularity. In: *Language, brain, and cognitive development*, ed. I. Dupoux, pp. 47–57. Cambridge, MA: MIT Press.

Sporns, O. (2015). Network neuroscience. In: *The future of the brain*, eds. G. Marcus & J. Freeman, pp. 90–99. Princeton: Princeton University Press.

Stanley, M. L., & De Brigard, F. (2016). Modularity in network neuroscience and neural reuse. *Behavioral and Brain Sciences, 39*, 29–31.

Stanton, N. A., & Salmon, P. M. (2009). Human error taxonomies applied to driving: A generic error taxonomy and its implications for intelligent transport systems. *Safety Science, 47*(2), 227–237.

Sterelny, K. (2006). Language, modularity, and evolution. In: *Teleosemantics*, eds. G. Macdonald & D. Papineau, pp. 23–41. Oxford: Oxford University Press.

Sterelny, K. (2012). *The evolved apprentice*. Cambridge, MA: MIT Press.

Sternberg, S. (2011). Modular processes in mind and brain. *Cognitive Neuropsychology, 28*(3–4), 156–208.

Striem-Amit, E., Dakwar, O., Reich, L., & Amedi, A. (2012). The large-scale organization of "visual" streams emerges without visual experience. *Cerebral Cortex, 22*(7), 1698–1709.

Striem-Amit, E., & Amedi, A. (2014). Visual cortex extrastriate body-selective area activation in congenitally blind people "seeing" by using sounds. *Current Biology, 24*, 1–6.

Suddendorf, T. (2013). *The gap: The science of what separates us from the animals*. New York: Basic Books.

Teyler, T. J. (2001). LTP and the superfamily of synaptic plasticities. In: *Toward a theory of neuroplasticity*, eds. C. A. Shaw & J. C. McEachern, pp. 101–117. Philadelphia: Psychology Press.

Thoenissen, D., Zilles, K., & Toni, I. (2002). Differential involvement of parietal and precentral regions in movement preparation and motor intention. *Journal of Neuroscience, 22*, 9024–9034.

van Gelder, T. (1995). What might cognition be, if not computation? *Journal of Philosophy, 92*(7), 345–381.

Varley, R. A., Klessinger, N. J. C., Romanowski, C. A. J., & Siegal, M. (2005). Agrammatic but numerate. *Proceedings of the National Academy of Sciences of the United States of America, 102*, 3519–3524.

Verhage, M., Maia, A. S., Plomp, J. J., Brussaard, A. B., Heeroma, J. H., Vermeer, H., Toonen, R. F., Hammer, R. E., van den Berg, T. K., Missler, M., Geuze, H. J., & Südhof, T. C. (2000). Synaptic assembly of the brain in the absence of neurotransmitter secretion. *Science, 287*(5454), 864–869.

Waddington, C. H. (1953). Genetic assimilation of an acquired character. *Evolution, 17*, 118–126.

Waddington, C. H. (1955). On a case of quantitative variation on either side of the wild type. *Molecular Genetics and Genomics,87*(2), 208–228.

Walker, G. H., Stanton, N. A., & Salmon, P. M. (2015). *Human factors in automotive engineering and technology*. Surrey: Ashgate.

Wernicke, C. (1908). The symptom-complex of aphasia. In: *Diseases of the nervous system*, ed. A. Church, pp. 265–324. New York: Appleton.

Whiteacre, J. M. (2010). Degeneracy: A link between evolvability, robustness and complexity in biological systems. *Theoretical Biology and Medical Modelling, 7*(6), 1–17.

Wolbers, T., Zahorik, P., & Giudice, N. A. (2011). Decoding the direction of auditory motion in blind humans. *NeuroImage, 56*(2), 681–687.

Wolpert, L. (2011). *Developmental biology: A very short introduction*. New York: Oxford University Press.

Zador, A. (2015). The connectome as a DNA sequencing problem. In: *The future of the brain*, eds. G. Marcus & J. Freeman, pp. 40–49. Princeton: Princeton University Press.

Zerilli, J. (2014). A minimalist framework for comparative psychology. *Biology and Philosophy, 29*(6), 897–904.

Zerilli, J. (2019). Multiple realization and the commensurability of taxonomies. *Synthese, 196*(8), 3337–3353.

Index

For the benefit of digital users, indexed terms that span two pages (e.g., 52– 53) may, on occasion, appear on only one of those pages.